Zero
BALANCING

Conscious Touch and Transformation

Praise for Zero Balancing

Reading Jim McCormick's book is a transformative experience itself. This delightfully written book, full of Zero Balancing client experiences, covers everything from ZB's theoretical basis to its principles, insight, and inspiration. It also explores the most important qualities in a healthy life as they happen between a practitioner and client. Jim demonstrates through his transparent and vulnerable writing how to be present with your whole self, whether writing a book or being in loving connection with a client on the table. I strongly recommend this book to every body-oriented therapist and every client wanting insight into the mind and heart of a master practitioner.

Ben E Benjamin PhD, President, Benjamin Institute. Author of *Listen to your Pain*

Whether you have no prior knowledge of Zero Balancing or years of experience, Jim McCormick's teaching and writing is like Mozart's music – you can whistle the tune, but also find endless depth and beauty there – in this testament to human potential. Jim shows in this important book, with remarkable clarity, how humans are capable of transformation. In this world, which deeply needs health, unity, and compassion, Jim singularly illuminates how Zero Balancing is a revelation for health practitioners, for receivers, and for everyone wanting to understand how to be at peace within ourselves, with each other, and with the world around us.

Not only through touch, but by placing this important book in our hands, Jim McCormick gives us the opportunity to see how Zero Balancing affects the very foundations of our structure and energy. Jim has a remarkable ability to clearly show how - with heart, touch, mind and a few well-placed words – Zero Balancing can uniquely help people to access the deepest places within their own energy and structure.

David Lauterstein author *The Deep Massage Book* and Co-director, Lauterstein-Conway Massage School

There are many hundreds of books that explain theories and techniques of holistic mind/body therapies. But this book is the only one I have come across that uses case studies primarily to illuminate the relationship of structure and energy in healing. In this sense it is unique and valuable to a wide range of people, not just Zero Balancers.

I think that the power of Zero Balancing for transformative healing comes from the power of touch. This book is a resource for expanding an awareness of touch as an important social as well as therapeutic beneficence.

David Laden Certified Zero Balancer, Advanced Certified Rolfer

In *Zero Balancing – conscious touch and transformation* Jim McCormick provides intriguing case studies and outlines clearly key principles for creating therapeutic relationships and connections through touch. The book will be attractive to anyone interested in healing, body-mind therapy, therapeutic touch, human potential and energy systems. The language and ideas are accessible for anyone who is interested in healing, and the book is full of insights for practitioners.

Amanda King Licensed Massage Therapist, Zero Balancing Instructor

Zero
BALANCING

Conscious Touch and Transformation

James McCormick

Forewords
Fritz Frederick Smith
James L Oschman

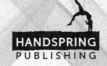

HANDSPRING
PUBLISHING

HANDSPRING PUBLISHING LIMITED
The Old Manse, Fountainhall,
Pencaitland, East Lothian
EH34 5EY, Scotland
Tel: +44 1875 341 859
Website: www.handspringpublishing.com
First published 2021 in the United Kingdom by Handspring Publishing
Copyright © Handspring Publishing 2021

ISBN 978-1-913426-15-6
ISBN (Kindle eBook) 978-1-913426-16-3

British Library Cataloguing in Publication Data
A catalogue record for this book is available from the British Library
Library of Congress Cataloguing in Publication Data
A catalog record for this book is available from the Library of Congress

Notice

Commissioning Editor: Mary Law
Project Manager: Morven Dean
Copy Editor: Glenys Norquay
Designer: Kirsteen Wright
Indexer: Aptara, India
Typesetter: DSM, India
Printer: CPI Group (UK) Ltd, Croydon, CR0 4YY

The Publisher's policy is to use paper manufactured from sustainable forests

Dedication

This book is dedicated to my major teachers, Dr Fritz Frederick Smith, Dr J.R. Worlsey, Dr Jorge Carballo; Dr Pamela Geib, my editor Michelle Blake, and most of all to my wife, Dr Betsy Kelly McCormick.

Contents

Contents

Foreword by Fritz Frederick Smith

Zero Balancing: Conscious Touch and Transformation is a multi-faceted yet very personal book. Jim McCormick articulates the fundamental principles of Zero Balancing, illustrating them with relevant case histories. While doing this he additionally describes the actual underlying processes of performing a Zero Balancing session. The book then becomes personal as he shares his own feelings, struggles and thoughts that occur for him during the performance of sessions. This personal flavor along with the multiple case reviews provides the reader with doorways for their own growth and transformation. I know I had a number of moments as I read Jim's book when I felt I was not only understanding the theory and process of ZB but was actually getting a session. I believe any Zero Balancing practitioner will gain meaningful insights from reading *Zero Balancing: Conscious Touch and Transformation*, and that any non-Zero Balancer will want a ZB session.

Fritz Frederick Smith, MD
Founder of Zero Balancing
February 2021

Foreword by
James L Oschman

In this fascinating book, James McCormick documents the wide range of transformative experiences that can emerge from a Zero Balancing session. I believe part of the reason for this variety is that every person presents with their own unique history of physical, emotional, and/or spiritual traumas. The overriding message is that these traumas compromise both body structure and energetics and can be resolved through this remarkably gentle process. By bringing physical and psycho-spiritual lives into harmony, a person is left with nothing but their own personal inner comfort. For me, Zero Balancing took me to a state of total bliss; a new and unanticipated experience. I realized that this is a rare state – most of us go through our lives without knowing the possibility that such a wonderful inner state even exists. It is delicious when it happens. Practitioners from every modality and from every level of expertise will find inspiration in the experiences and insights James documents here. For those who have yet to experience Zero Balancing, the book will give you insights about this remarkably effective method of feeling completely at home.

James L. Oschman, PhD
Author of *Energy Medicine: The Scientific Basis*
March 2021

Preface

Hello Darkness, My Old Friend

In March 2016, Dr Fritz Smith, came to the Boston area to teach a new class he had just created, called Zero Balancing and Consciousness. Fritz, at 92, is still actively teaching and learning. This particular class was about how to work with consciousness through Zero Balancing. That is, how to help guide the client into deeper, altered states of consciousness where more change is possible, not only in her body but also in her awareness. The session I describe below happened in my office a day after that class.

Ella works in corporate America and has received ZB sessions for several years. She has also taken a number of ZB classes herself. She receives ZB from me every few months. Her goal for this session was, "I just want to have a wonderful ZB session – without limiting the possibilities by having some specific want." Sometimes we say to a client, "Let's have a session that serves your highest good," without needing to be specific about what that would be, and trusting that it can happen. Her wish was similar to that idea.

I used some of the fulcrums that Fritz had just taught to help move her into an altered state of consciousness, where she could become more connected to her deepest core self. (We use the word fulcrum in Zero Balancing to mean any time we touch the body. We create a fulcrum in many ways, such as lifting, bending, pulling, twisting or compressing. The fulcrum is designed to make a change in the client's system.)

Often when a client has gone to a deep state quickly, there is the possibility of overload – of doing more than the person can integrate easily or well. In this case I decided it was safe to do as much as Ella could tolerate, and to watch her carefully to make sure I didn't overdo it. This is always a clinical judgment, but Ella is experienced with Zero Balancing, and I was confident that she would respond well to stronger work. It turned out that Ella was fine with it all, continuing to have full, deep breaths and to get quieter in her body, and yet also feeling more alive. Ella's bones and the soft tissues literally felt livelier, more elastic, and more vibrant, and similarly her energetic field became more lively and sparkly. And in between these movements she would have periods of extreme stillness, her body not moving while her energetic field grew quieter and quieter.

During an altered state the client's awareness goes inside her body as she is paying more attention to the shifts she is feeling in her body, mind and spirit on the inside. She is less attuned to the outside world. For many reasons we will discuss later, this allows more change in the client in both amount of energy, in feelings and often in bodily symptoms. This process is observable to the Zero Balancer and was clearly happening with Ella.

At the end of the session, Ella took a while coming out of the experience after I had taken my hands off. She stayed very still with her eyes closed for a long time. Only then did she begin to show emotion. During that time a few tears began to drip from her eyes. She opened her eyes, and as we began to talk about her experience, the

Fulcrums

In Zero Balancing the fulcrum is our working tool. A fulcrum is a specific field of tension that we create through touch. Any held field of tension can create a fulcrum: lifting, bending, sliding, pushing, pulling, twisting, compressing. A fulcrum serves as a catalyst to promote change and is itself not affected by the action.

There are three, sometimes overlapping classes of fulcrums.

1. **Point of reference fulcrums:**

    These fulcrums act by being held stationary for short periods of time (from 1 to 7 seconds) and promote balance and local change. They are represented by:

    *   Simple lifting fulcrums, as used on the ribs.
    *   Constructed fulcrums which, when held stationary, can act as a point, as seen with the hip fulcrum.

2. **Field fulcrums:**

    These fulcrums place a clearer, stronger vibration through an area of the body, releasing or influencing the weaker vibration. These fulcrums can be created with a straight pull, a curved pull, or with compression.

    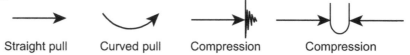

    | Straight pull | Curved pull | Compression | Compression |

    With a straight pull, all the tension moves in one direction. With a curved pull, there are an infinite number of tangents. Use a curved fulcrum to address a curved structure.

    In ZB we refer to the curved pull as a half moon vector (HMV), in that it has both a magnitude and a direction, and is in the form of a crescent (as represented by a half moon).

    The half moon vector is a hallmark fulcrum of Zero Balancing. It is used in a number of places during a ZB session: through the legs, neck, tarsal bones, and closing fulcrums.

    The half moon vector has a number of uses. It can orient a person to themselves; create clearer, stronger fields in the body: and integrate work that has been done.

    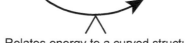

    Relates energy to a curved structure

3. **Moving fulcrums:**

    These fulcrums are characterized by using the client's own energy to create a bolus and move it through their own tissue. Examples of this are: the lateral leg sweep, HMV with a twist using the second hand on the neck, the suboccipital sweep (SOS).

    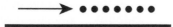

Different Types of Fulcrums used in Zero Balancing.

(Illustrations by Fritz Smith, used with permission of the Zero Balancing Touch Foundation.)

first thing she said was she felt sad. She was crying slightly and then soon after smiling and laughing.

We talked for thirty minutes after the session, longer than in most appointments. She was very animated during this time. She looked, and said she felt, totally alive. She had a beautiful expression of amazement on her face at the experience she'd just had.

She talked about the rhythm of the session, saying the fulcrums and the pauses were perfect. She was having images of her ex-partner as a young man, and seeing younger and younger images of him as the session went on. There was a lot of sadness with these images. I had done one fulcrum where I gently held her head with great care and connection and asked her to just let her head rest in my hands. She felt a huge "whoosh of sadness" during this fulcrum and after I took my hands off of her head.

Ella often hears music in her head during a ZB session and this time the music was "The Sound of Silence," from Simon and Garfunkel. "Hello darkness, my old friend; I've come to talk with you again," which connected her back to the loss she had suffered in that relationship. The "whoosh," and the pause after, allowed her to feel those feelings of sadness deeply, but then to move through them to other feelings. The sadness was not repressed at that point, but fully experienced and transcended.

As we talked further she said she felt "refreshed and renewed… I feel alive like I haven't felt for decades… I can't stop smiling. I feel so much joy it's almost bursting out of me… I feel new… I feel surprised… I feel like dancing… I have a swagger to me."

As she felt this joy, she began to connect to her younger self who, she remembered, was "smiling all the time." She even remembered a woman she worked with who told her to "stop smiling all the time." She had felt so alive and happy at that time and remarked, "It's been so long since I felt that way." She began to feel totally connected to her own younger self and so delighted to be connected again. There are many techniques for asking a client to dialogue with her inner child. I asked Ella to speak to her younger self and tell that self how happy she was to be in touch with her again. This connection made her younger self (and her current adult self) extremely happy.

As we talked further, Ella's tone began to change again. She realized she had felt really good in herself when she met her former partner and not so good after. She was still feeling the joy in this moment and at the same time feeling sadness for having been away from this joy for so long. This experience is called mourning the self. Often after someone has made a big breakthrough in her personal work, and is feeling the delight and expansiveness of this new place, she can begin to feel sad at not having been in this place earlier in her life. She can become aware of all the opportunities she missed by not being able to access the joy and openness during those years. Even though there is sadness involved, from the practitioner's point of view, this is a very healthy and important part of the process and indicates deep movement has happened for the person. Ella went into the sadness for a while, and we talked about it, and then she was able to transition back to the joy.

This is a great example of what I mean by a transformational session. A different person came off the table than the one who started out on the table. These are often watershed moments for the client. Clients tend to remember these experiences for a long time, and often refer back to them as the time when their lives changed.

The lesson for me from this session was that I pushed the envelope – kept doing deeper fulcrums even after there had already been a lot of change. And in this case it led to a groundbreaking personal change for Ella.

A few days later I wrote to check in with her and received this reply:

Hi, Jim,

I was thinking of sending you an email when I got out of work tonight, and I got one from you!

Monday's session was momentous. It really felt like something major opened up inside for me. I didn't want to go home right away so I had a quick dinner at S&S Deli. And flirted with a young guy on my way out! That young and carefree girl just sprung out before I could stop her! I meditated a little after I got home but it was difficult to sit still, so I gave up after less than 10 minutes and just walked around a little, with a swagger of course. The sleep Monday night was totally peaceful.

Unfortunately, my work schedule was jam-packed yesterday and today. I could sense the light around me dimming as things started to pile up. The good news is that I seem to be able to cope better just by sinking into my body and "feel/be more present". That's another term that I heard many times from you but didn't really grasp the meaning until now.

Thank you again for another wonderful ZB session. I am truly grateful for everything you have done for me.

Ella

A session with a very different client, Doug, reveals another way that transformation can occur in Zero Balancing, for the client and the practitioner. Doug is a 45-year-old engineer in good health who came in for a ZB session many years ago. During our initial discussion, his goal for the session emerged: "I want you to help me remove my doubt." This session turned out to be a major milestone in the depth of my work with Zero Balancing.

Doug didn't specify exactly what doubt he wanted to get rid of. He was not open to doing a lot of talking about it. When he stated his intention, I immediately had a lot of doubt. Could I deliver on that request? Was Zero Balancing really able to help people in that way? I hadn't done this before. I debated internally whether to accept this as the goal for the session, and finally decided to go ahead.

I began the session doing an evaluation with Doug sitting on the table, and as I palpated his upper back and shoulders what I found was unremarkable. I certainly had no clue at this point about how to help his doubts. Nonetheless, I had him lie down and went to his feet to start the session with what we call a half moon vector (a curved pull through the legs to engage the whole body). As I held his feet and lifted his legs, I was astonished. I began to sense energy pockets or patterns within his energy field that were different from his overall energy.

In Zero Balancing we like to say that each of us has two bodies. Each person has a physical body and also has an energy body. In Zero Balancing we want to connect to both of those parts of the person. And particularly we want to be able to perceive the energy body of the client – both with our touch and with our eyes. It is possible both to touch the energy body and to see it.

I often see the energy field of a client with patterns that look like the silvery, shimmering light of the moon on the sea at night. With Doug I saw, in his energetic field, areas that were light and bright and other areas that were darker and less clear. It struck me that these darker areas might be the areas of doubt. As I went through the Zero Balancing protocol working with the whole body, I felt many such areas.

Since this was a new experience, I wasn't sure what to do, but I decided to act as if these denser,

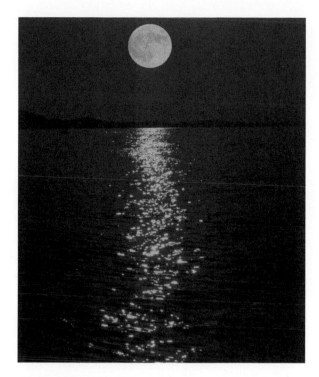

Shimmering Light of the moon on the sea at night.

(Photo: Shutterstock.)

different areas were in fact where his doubt was residing as held energy, both in his body/mind and in his energy field. When I placed Zero Balancing fulcrums in these areas, the quality of the patterns changed. The difference between these areas and other areas of the body lessened. The whole field felt smoother and more congruent and coherent, more uniformly lit up.

By the time I finished we hadn't said a word, but I felt his system was much easier and more integrated. He felt lighter and clearer. He later reported that over the next days he continued to feel stronger and to experience less doubt.

What was most remarkable about the session was not so much this particular outcome, but the learning I experienced from doing the session. From that day forward I started to pay more attention to the quality of the feelings that appeared in the imbalances and the blockages I found in people's bodies. If I palpated a place of held or blocked energy in someone's body, I explored more deeply and with more curiosity into the sensation. I paid careful attention to that place of held energy without trying to change it. I would do my best to just be with it. I would ask myself "What is the emotion or sensation being held here"? I learned that I could identify any emotion or sensation in the body because they all had different vibratory signatures. Each emotion or sensation had a particular energetic signature that was unique, and I could learn to feel it and identify it.

Fear has a very different vibratory quality than anger or joy or grief. Initially I started paying attention to the major emotions (fear, grief, anger, joy) as they were the strongest and clearest, and therefore the easiest to feel. Sometimes this opened up a whole new avenue of healing for the person by identifying a feeling he wasn't aware of. I might say, "I can feel a sensation in your body which I think is fear. Are you feeling afraid"? One of the first clients I said that to replied, "Only a mountain of it." This led to a huge outpouring of feeling and tears from her. We had a long conversation we'd never had before about her fears, and this in turn led to major changes, not only for that session, but also for her choices in her life.

Through gradually exploring the expression of emotions in the body, I learned I could feel, in the physical body, what was happening for the person. The possibility of verbally processing emotions discovered through the body/mind connection opened much deeper possibilities of healing and change, and the discoveries led me to work in very different ways.

For instance, I now teach students how to feel these vibrations in their clients. They can most easily learn to feel the main emotions, but once they have success in feeling those emotions they quickly learn they can feel other emotions (like anxiety or depression). If someone has feelings of indecision, agitation, indifference, guilt, lack of motivation or any other emotional quality, these sensations show up in the energetic field and can be identified through touch. The practitioner can then work with them.

For me, this often means continuing to do the Zero Balancing, but with a different quality to my touch. Not only can I "read" an emotion in someone through my hands, but also I can offer an emotion with my hands. I might touch with the same quality I would use if I were to pick up a small, frightened child I wanted to comfort. I would hold the child in such a way that he felt safe, secure and reassured. So for an adult client with fear, I do the fulcrums with that quality of touch, and find that it creates much greater positive change. Clients with major fears calm down, without me ever saying anything to them about their fear.

This is true not only for fear, but for any emotion or sensation. I learned over time that through touch, often without even talking about it, I could help make major shifts in the emotional life of many clients, in addition to the physical shifts that Zero Balancing can generate. This can often lead to deep personal change, and is part of what makes Zero Balancing a transformational tool. The clients begin to feel they are more alive, more vital and more at home in themselves.

James McCormick
Cambridge, Massachusetts, USA
February 2021

Acknowledgments

I have had huge help in many different ways from many different people. More than I can list here. But I specifically want to thank these people who have had major input into the book and into helping me get all the way to the finish.

First of all, Mary Law and the people of Handspring Publishing, including Morven Dean. Hillary Brown, Stephanie Ricks, Fiona Conn, and Glenys Norquay, have been wonderful to work with. They have been helpful, supportive and patient. I am grateful to them for getting this book published and in the right venue.

Michelle Blake for being a sterling editor helping my writing become much better and much easier to read. And for her unflagging encouragement. Without her I could easily have stopped at many different times. She had faith in me and in this project. I am especially grateful to her.

Lucy Lopez for huge help with formatting much of the book to help me get it ready for final publication.

Misty Rhoads and Mary Murphy for huge editing help and encouragement. They were both instrumental in helping me over some rough spots. They gave me great feedback when I needed it. And they were both willing to have their work included in the research chapter in this book.

Thanks so much to James Strickland and Stuart Reynolds of the Neuro Synchrony Institute in Austin for their help with research into the effects of Zero Balancing and the understanding of the research in general. They were fantastic to work with.

Special thanks to Fritz Smith for all of his love, support, teaching and friendship over many years, and for writing a Foreword for this book; and to Jim Oschman both for his Foreword and for his support of energy medicine for many years.

Amanda King for huge help with pictures and always believing in me and this project. David Laden was also tremendous with his comments and support.

The Board of the Zero Balancing Touch Foundation for their support of this project and the use of materials from the Zero Balancing Study Guide.

Jessica Kern, Eliza Mallouk, David Laden. Michele Doucette, James Salomons and Jackie Eve for reviewing and commenting on the manuscript.

Deanne Waggy and Tom Gentile for providing numerous pictures.

My wife, Betsy Kelly McCormick, has been a huge and steady base of support and encouragement throughout the whole process. Without her it never would have happened.

James McCormick
Cambridge, Massachusetts, USA
February 2021

About the Author

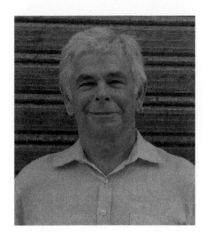

James McCormick, LAc., began his study of Traditional Chinese Acupuncture in 1972 in England. He was introduced to Zero Balancing in 1974, and has been practicing ZB ever since and became the first teacher of Zero Balancing after Dr Fritz Smith, the founder.

He recently retired after fifteen years as president of the Zero Balancing Touch Foundation, a non-profit foundation designed to support Zero Balancing and conscious touch modalities worldwide, and to conduct research on and support educational conferences on the same topics.

He is co-director of Cambridge Health Associates, a holistic health center in Cambridge, MA, practicing both Five Element Acupuncture and Zero Balancing.

He lives in Wayland, Massachusetts, with his wife.

Glossary

AEDP: Accelerated Experiential Dynamic Psychotherapy, a form of psychotherapy developed by Dr Diana Fosha.

Altered states of consciousness: Refers to any state of awareness outside our normal waking consciousness.

Amplify: In ZB, a term that refers to fulcrums whose main intent is to increase the strength of the energy field in the client.

Bones: In ZB, the primary area where the Zero Balancer is applying the fulcrums (because we believe the bones carry the strongest energy fields in the body and that tension stored in the bones often holds unprocessed information and early conditioning patterns).

Borborygmus: A rumbling or gurgling noise made by the movement of fluid and gas in the intestines.

Deep breaths: One of the working signs of energy movement in the body. See working signs, under working state.

Donkey touch: The term used in Zero Balancing for when the practitioner consciously touches both the structure and energy of the client. (This type of touch often leads to the client feeling deeply met and reacting to the touch from a more instinctual, as opposed to a mental, place.)

Emotional signatures in the body: As we all know there are many varieties of each emotion. There are as many types of fear as there are colors of water in the ocean. There is terror; there is apprehension, shyness, anxiety, trembling and stage fright, to name a few. Each feels different both to the person experiencing them and to the Zero Balancer feeling them in the client's body. Yet, they all have something in common and feel very different from anger or grief. The vibration of fear often has a shaky or quaky quality in the tissue.

Anger has a different signature. As with fear, there are as many kinds of anger as there are greens on the trees. There is anger, rage, irritation, annoyance, frustration, stubbornness, resistance, jealousy and others. And even when we use the same word, there are many types of rage and many types of irritation. So the list of words that describe what anger (or any emotion) feels like is varied and only some of them will apply to each person's anger. Nonetheless there are some similarities among these sensations, so they feel more like one another than they do like grief or fear. In ancient China, acupuncturists had a description of the feeling in an angry person's pulse – "this feels like a taut guitar string." These descriptions are all different from the words we used above to describe fear.

The feeling of joy or happiness is even more distinct. A person feeling joy has tissues and energetic fields that feel light, expansive, inviting, flowing, free, inspiring.

Grief is thinner, more brittle, more pulled in (meaning pulled away from the external); it can be hard also but a different hardness from anger, more dull or without a lot of vibration.

Energy: The energy felt in the body; synonyms for energy include: vibration, movement, wave, force, tension, vitality.

Expanded consciousness: See Altered states of consciousness.

Foundation joints: A set of joints in the body that have as their major function the transmission of energy rather than movement of locomotion; also a small range of motion and no voluntary muscles over these joints. They include the cranial sutures, the sacroiliac joint, the tarsal joints of the feet and the carpal bones of the hands.

Framing: A clear agreement with the ZB client stating the aims of a ZB session or group of sessions. This clarity for both the client and the practitioner often allows more change to happen.

Fulcrum: In ZB, our basic working tool of touch. A fulcrum is a specific field of tension created by lifting, bending, sliding, pushing, pulling or twisting.

Interface: The desired touch used in Zero Balancing; a form of touch that creates a clear boundary between the client and the practitioner, in which both know where one's body/energy ends and the other's body/energy begins, created when the practitioner keeps his awareness on the place where his fingers meet the body of the client. This awareness helps to create the clear boundary.

Protocol: The term used for the format of a typical Zero Balancing session.

Structure: In ZB, the word used to reference all aspects of the physical body.

Working state: The period when the client is integrating energy and structure and her body/mind is shifting. This state often causes a number of body signs indicating a shift, and may also indicate an expanded state of consciousness. These body signs are called the working signs. These signs can be used to monitor a client's progress during a session and include watching the eyes and the breath and listening to the voice vitality.

Zero balancing: A hands-on body/mind system of therapy designed to enhance health by balancing body structure with body energy.

Introduction

My experience with Zero Balancing began when I was 26 years old. I had just finished two years as a conscientious objector to the Vietnam War working at a human potential growth center in Concord, Massachusetts, The Associates for Human Resources. This was a group of psychotherapists, psychologists and educators who worked in the fields of organizational development and personal development. The first time I met them, I was amazed and impressed by how carefully they spoke and listened to one another. They were determined to be understood and to understand what the other was saying.

I spent two years attending various encounter groups of all types, and doing my first psychotherapeutic work. That experience created a major shift in my life from being a left brain, linear thinker (math and physics major in undergraduate school) to a more balanced human being, accessing more of my right brain and my emotions. This changed my life for the better, allowing me access to all of my self. In addition, I learned about energy in the body as opposed to the energy talked about in physics (e=mc²). This included studies in various forms of energy therapy, specifically Bio-energetic Psychotherapy and Gestalt Therapy.

At that time, 1971, Richard Nixon made major news by visiting China. He was the first president to do so since 1949. This was a significant political event but also led to the introduction of acupuncture to the United States. James Reston, a columnist for the New York Times, had an emergency appendectomy in China with acupuncture as the anesthesia. It was successful, and when he returned and wrote about it, acupuncture hit America in a big way.

The European countries had not cut ties to Communist China as the US had, and acupuncture and other Eastern arts had flourished all through Europe in the 1950s and 1960s. In the fall of 1972 I went off to study acupuncture in England, in the first acupuncture class for Americans offered by Dr J.R. Worsley. We met in a hotel in Kenilworth, England. There were forty people in the class, mostly somewhat wild Americans, doing headstands in the lobby of the hotel where we stayed, and some people well-known or about to become well-known (including Hector Prestera; three people from the Arica studies of Oscar Ichazo; Harriet Beinfield, Efrem Korngold and Bob Duggan; Diane Connelly; Jack Daniel, and more). Dr Fritz Smith was part of that group.

Fritz was an osteopathic MD, with a full-time practice of osteopathy in Watsonville, California. In the late afternoons when acupuncture class was over he would work on our fellow students with his osteopathy skills, and I would follow him and watch. I learned so much, because he would describe what he was doing and point out what was changing in the person he was working with.

One day I sat next to him at lunch. To emphasize some point he was making he put his hand on my shoulder and the touch was so warm, clear and loving, I still remember it to this day.

That touch, plus watching him work, led me to ask Fritz to give me a Zero Balancing session.

It wasn't yet called Zero Balancing, but all the key parts of the work were there even in this early stage. As I said earlier, I was immediately aware of the profound effect ZB had on me and of my desire to help others with this tool.

As part of our acupuncture training we each had to do a "project of excellence" of some kind. Fritz decided to create a class to teach acupuncturists how to work with body structure. As he formulated the class he had many insights from our acupuncture learnings about the relationship between body energy and body structure, and these became incorporated in his teachings.

Once Fritz began teaching this work, I asked him to come to Boston. This was 1974, and the class was called "Functional Manipulation." I believe it was the second class he taught in this method. That began a long, deep mentoring relationship and friendship with Fritz, which exists to this day. Fritz was one of the first people in my life I felt I could fully trust because he "walked his talk."

I kept soaking up as much as I could, taking numerous classes and incorporating that work into my acupuncture practice. Zero Balancing and Traditional Five Element Acupuncture proved to be a beautiful match, and I have been pursuing their integration ever since. In 1979 I became the first teacher of Zero Balancing after Fritz, and when Zero Balancing certification began in 1982, I was proud to be the first person certified to practice Zero Balancing. Receiving, practicing and teaching Zero Balancing, along with my association with Fritz, has transformed my life and my work, making both aspects of my life more exciting and more inspired.

Zero Balancing is useful for many things including a range of physical complaints, from headaches to plantar fasciitis. We will look at these uses later in the book, but right now I want to focus on the use of Zero Balancing for personal transformation.

When I use the word "transformation," what do I mean? I mean the process of becoming more in touch with one's core self. There are some common experiences of being in touch with one's core: knowing and understanding one's self; being able to keep awareness in the present moment; and an experience of just "being" in which there is nothing to do. Finally, there is a feeling of joy and peace and a sense of well-being that does not depend on what happens in the outer world.

Another word for this process of transformation is self-actualization. Self-actualization is a term introduced by Kurt Goldstein in the 1930s and 1940s and used later by many others, particularly by Abraham Maslow in the area of humanistic psychology. In Goldstein's view: "The tendency to actualize one's self as fully as possible is the basic human drive." Another way he described self-actualization was the "full realization of one's talents and potentialities."

Maslow agreed and said there is a hierarchy of needs in life: "1) the physiological needs for air and food; 2) safety; 3) belonging and love; 4) self-esteem, self-respect, and healthy positive feelings; 5) and the being needs – concerning creative self-growth engendered from fulfillment of potential and meaning in life." (Maslow, 1943) He said self-actualization represents the "growth of an individual toward fulfilling the highest needs in this hierarchy" – those for "meaning in life" and for "being." His belief was that "finding your core-nature that is unique to you is one of the main goals of life." The quest for spiritual enlightenment, the pursuit of knowledge and a desire to transform society are other examples of self-actualization or personal transformation.

Diana Fosha, the founder of Accelerated Experiential Dynamic Psychotherapy (AEDP), has created her own list of some of the qualities

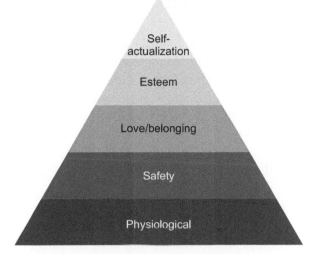

Maslow – hierarchy of needs. (See en.wikipedia.org/wiki/Self-actualization)

(Originally published in Maslow A (1943) A theory of human motivation, *Psychological Review* 50, 370–96.)

of a self-actualized person: "Calm, flow, ease, compassion, curiosity, creativity and clarity, where the sense of truth comes from deep acceptance and self-acceptance." In AEDP there is a view that we are all wired for what she calls "transformance," the idea that there is an innate drive in everyone to grow, to evolve and to self-actualize. In the AEDP literature they talk about someone who is living in that self-actualized place as being in touch with her "self at best" or "true self."

There are many paths to self-development including meditation, psychotherapy, prayer and yoga. In the general public, if people have heard of ZB at all, they tend to think of it as beneficial for relaxation and certain physical complaints. What is much less widely known is that Zero Balancing can play an important role in the development of personal growth and transformation.

Over time, Zero Balancing helps clients to live more from that place of harmony. Through touch, Zero Balancing can help introduce a client

Advantages of Zero Balancing

Zero Balancing has elements of all of the disciplines mentioned above, but Zero Balancing has several advantages:

1. Zero Balancing adds the element of touch, which can speed up this process tremendously. Through touch you can often help place the person in a deep meditative state, with a profound connection to his core self in a matter of minutes.

2. ZB works directly with the body and with a part of the body (the bones) that gives direct access to the core of the person.

3. ZB is very good at reducing or removing the blocks in our bodies that make it harder to connect with the true self, thus allowing easier access to deeper parts of the self.

4. All of this helps keep the person's awareness in the present moment. What's happening in the body is happening now. This is one of the main teachings of all spiritual traditions. When the client can pay attention to what's happening in her body, she can keep her focus on what is real and current and not on fears or regrets, which are in the future or the past.

to her core self, and she can then return there more easily on her own.

Alan Hext, a Zero Balancing teacher from the United Kingdom, likes to say that ZB is a "classic," in the sense that its principles are based on

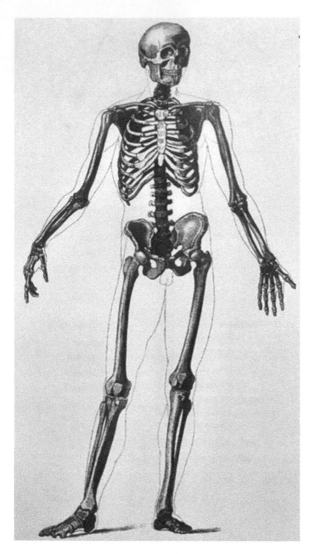

In Zero Balancing we focus our attention mainly on the bones and the skeletal system.

(Photo: James McCormick.)

nature and thus are timeless. Zero Balancing practitioners and teachers think ZB has universal application for healing through touch, as well as universal principles to follow for a full life. I believe that to be true, and I think it is one of

many ways that ZB can make a positive contribution to our world.

A typical Zero Balancing session lasts 30–40 minutes and is done with the client fully clothed and lying down on a massage table. The Zero Balancer (ZBer) will frequently start with the client sitting up and will evaluate certain parts of the client's body while the client is sitting and then have the client lie down. The bodywork starts with the lower body, moves to the upper body and finishes by returning to the lower body.

In each area, the Zero Balancing practitioner evaluates the movement of energy through the bones and joints, reading both the range of motion and the quality of the energy moving through the bones and soft tissue, especially the ligaments. When imbalances are found, the practitioner uses gentle pressure, traction and rotation to bring about increased motion in both the physical body and the energy body.

A Zero Balancing session generally feels extremely pleasurable to the client and leaves her feeling more relaxed and less anxious. In a research project on the effects of Zero Balancing, done in 2017 in Austin, Texas, through the Neuro Synchrony Institute, there was on average a 61% reduction in anxiety, stress and tension (which means that many people had even greater improvement). Both the Zero Balancers and the clients were measured on six different physiological scales. The measurements obtained from these readings correlated well with the subjective replies to a questionnaire completed by the subjects. You can get more information on this study by visiting the website of the Zero Balancing Touch Foundation, zbtouch.org, and clicking on the Research tab.

Let me give you a brief overview of the book:

It begins with two case histories without a lot of theory, to let the reader dive right into the

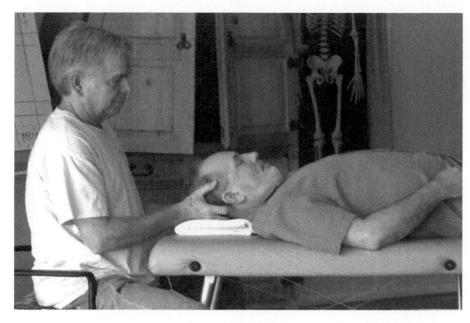

Author doing Zero Balancing on the upper body

(Photo: Tom Gentile.)

experience of Zero Balancing. Each chapter in Part One (Basic Principles of Zero Balancing) describes one of the basic principles of Zero Balancing practice and also illustrates that principle through one or more case studies of Zero Balancing sessions. Part Two (Healing Principles) is a more general discussion of healing principles that are widely applicable to Zero Balancing and beyond, also illustrated by appropriate ZB case studies. Part Three (Body, Mind, and Spirit) is a description of a series of ZB sessions with the same person, in order to give a better idea of how ZB works over time. These sessions

began in response to a physical need, but led to a transformation of a much deeper sort. Part Four (Transformation) is a description of a client's experience of her Zero Balancing session followed by my describing my experience of the same session. Part Five (Research on Zero Balancing) presents the current state of research into Zero Balancing.

Certain words as I go along may be unfamiliar to the reader, at least in the contexts in which I use them. I will define some of these words where they occur, and others can be found in the Glossary.

Part One

Basic Principles of Zero Balancing

Chapter 1
A Skittish Donkey

One of the joys of either giving or receiving Zero Balancing (ZB) is observing the absolute unity of the body, the mind and the spirit, and seeing this manifest over and over again. One of the most common questions I ask clients, especially those who are a bit lost or a bit out of touch with their own experience is, "If you pay attention to your body, without trying to change anything, what do you notice?" The mere act of beginning to notice what they feel in their bodies, especially if done without judgment, will cause changes in how they perceive themselves and the world around them. Physical pains will often diminish. Anxiety, fear, anger and depression will often begin to lessen when the client listens to her internal experience.

This session is a good example of how Zero Balancing can work with this incredible unity of mind, body and spirit to help the client feel her own strength and resilience. Carol, a 60-year-old woman with a lot of experience with ZB, came for a session. As we talked I kept thinking, "What is really the issue here? What is the main thing she needs?" I wasn't getting any hint. It was as if no useful information was being released. I experienced her as very defended. She did not want to be seen.

All of sudden I heard her say, "I feel like I've lost connection to myself." This perked me up. She was getting in touch with a real part of her experience (of not feeling in touch with herself), but at the same time she was letting herself be seen. She was letting me see that she felt lost and out of touch. She was making herself vulnerable, and for me that was the key to helping her move from that place.

Carol started talking about how her heart felt at this time, as if it had a very hard shell around it. This was an image she'd had since early in childhood. As she talked, it was easy to see from her history that the shell was needed when she was young, in order to protect her heart. But it was not just an image. As we explored, we found a real area of hardness, literally, in her chest. She felt the hardness but not much other sensation in that part of her body.

Our goals for the session became to help her feel connected to herself, to see if that hardness in her chest could soften and, if so, find out what would appear there instead. We began the session. I immediately put both hands on her shins and just listened with my hands. Could I feel connected to her through touch? If so, what did I feel? And could I help her get connected to herself?

I waited a long time without moving and without doing anything but resting my hands on her shins and paying attention to what I felt. I was waiting for her to show up, for her energy to show up.

We use the term *donkey* a lot in ZB. A little description now will help with understanding this case history and others. The term references the part of our bodies not under our conscious control – the unconscious, instinctual, animal part of us. It also represents our energy body, and is contrasted with *the rider*, which represents our minds. This is an important concept in ZB and is explained more fully later in the book, as well as in the glossary.

In this case I was waiting for her energy field, her *donkey*, to tell me it was ready for me to begin. As I waited, the information started to get clearer. I felt a *skittish donkey*. By that I mean that her clear core energy kept coming and going, peeking its head out and then going away. It was

like playing hide and seek with a young child. It felt as if she wanted to be connected and play but was very nervous about it. I stayed with that sensation while giving the donkey the message, non-verbally, that what it was doing was okay, and that I would wait until it was more steady and ready for me to go ahead.

I am not sure how long this took, maybe as long as a minute or two in clock time, which is much longer than usual. ZB fulcrums are often held for seconds, rather than minutes, so this was a special case.

Eventually I said out loud to her, "What I feel is a skittish donkey." She immediately laughed with recognition and was kind of delighted by the image. It took her back to one of her earliest and most common images for herself, which was a groundhog, or prairie dog, who would pop her head up to look around but then vanish into the hole at a moment's notice if danger arrived. We talked about this for a minute and laughed

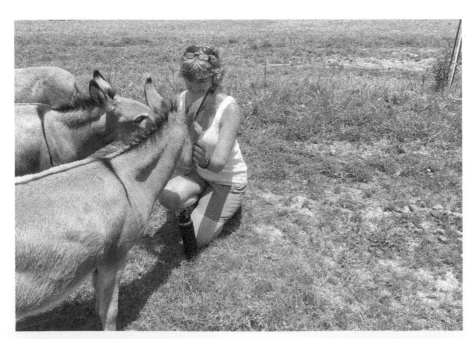

Fig. 1.1
Donkey – Metaphor for touching the instinctual response by touching energy and structure simultaneously and consciously.

(Photo: Ricardo Villa-lobos.)

about it. As we talked, the feeling under my hands changed a lot, and the skittishness lessened. It seemed that being seen and met allowed the donkey to feel safe to relax, to trust me to let the work happen.

We then went forward with the ZB, and at each place that I touched I paused a long time to wait for the donkey to indicate, "Okay, I'm ready now." I would initially not feel much, almost an absence of sensation, an absence of contact and an absence of movement. After a waiting period (while maintaining my connection as much as possible) there would be a deep breath, a sigh and a relaxation. This was always accompanied by a stronger sense of aliveness and energy under my hands. Suddenly there would be something to work with, as if someone had turned the water on, similar to the feeling of the Ch'i arriving at the acupuncture needle.

My mantra to myself for working with this client was, "Listen; go slow; wait for the donkey; hold the connection for as long as the body wants." This process allowed us to get more and more connected over time. Eventually I didn't need to wait at each place that I touched. The trust of her donkey had been earned. The connection had been made and didn't need to be re-established at each touch.

As I continued the ZB session, Carol began to have a series of images and sensations that were important to her and to me, and I think important to her ability to let go and connect more fully to herself, to me and to her life. When I held a fulcrum a long time on her right hip, with a deep connection, she clearly had some reaction. I didn't know what it was, but I began to feel tears in my eyes, so I asked, "What are you feeling now?"

She took a while answering, so I said, "I don't know about you, but I am feeling tears in my eyes." She immediately said, "Yes," and had a few tears. And then she said, "I feel sadness, and joy, and alive, all at the same time. It feels so exquisite."

As I moved to her upper back with steady, clear, patient touch, an image of a donkey also appeared to her. Her image was of a sure-footed, four-footed, sturdy, homely and stubborn donkey. I asked her "Are you feeling any of those qualities in you?" and she said, "Yes, especially surefooted. I feel like I have four strong hooves and it is not easy to push me over." I said I appreciated her strength and ability not to be pushed around (which is real) and suggested to her that this is among her strongest qualities and very different from her earlier skittishness.

Carol then had a dream-like image of being in the Grand Canyon and of a man trying to push a donkey off a cliff. In the fantasy, he couldn't do it. He could not push the donkey over the cliff. The donkey wouldn't move. The man had done this on purpose to reassure the people on the trail ride that the donkeys would not go off the cliff no matter what. You can try to push them off and they still won't go, so you don't have to fear falling off the trail. She started to feel that strength in herself, as well as a lessening of fear.

She also felt open and expansive. She was no longer the closed, lost person she had been at the beginning of the session. She began to have a desire to use her creative side. She felt a huge amount of energy building in her, and she wanted to use it. She wanted to do something and create something and she could feel the excitement building in her.

This led to her final image of being on a narrow trail in the Grand Canyon, now totally surefooted and with no fear. She felt solid and grounded and yet, at the same time, had the huge expanse of the canyon right there at her beck and call. She could enjoy this vast expansiveness and still be totally secure. We often call ZB a grounded high, and this client was experiencing that completely. She felt expanded and grounded at the same time. This was a joyous feeling for her.

She finished the session feeling that expansion, and yet still grounded and connected to herself. She was very happy, grateful, softer, more alive and happy. She appeared much more in touch with herself. She no longer seemed lost. In addition, she had softened the hard walnut shell around her heart. It felt literally softer and lighter in her chest – the physical hardness was gone. Her tissues had changed, mirroring the change in her psyche. This allowed her to feel joy, along with a connection to herself and to others.

Chapter 2
Structure and Energy: Listening for the Donkey

The definition of Zero Balancing is the art of simultaneously touching and balancing the structure and the energy of the body. In fact, it is often this experience of touching both energy and structure that makes a Zero Balancing session memorable, when the sensations and perceptions of the receiver are intensified and felt in the whole body. By the *structure* of the body, we mean the physical body – the bones, the organs, the muscles, skin and other soft tissue. Of course, our physical structure is vitally important to our health and much of medicine is devoted to healing this part of our being.

The *energy* part is a more difficult idea for some people to grasp. In Asian cultures the concept of Ch'i energy is better understood. Ch'i is central to all ancient Chinese practices – not just in medicine, but also in painting, poetry, music, dance, martial arts, politics, spirituality and, indeed, all of life. We know there are many energetic aspects of the body, including heat, electrical signals in the brain and body, electrons floating in our blood and lymph systems. All of these create electric fields.

Zero Balancers believe there is a bio-energy in the body, different from the nervous system, which influences the nervous system. If so, our scientific instruments are not yet sensitive enough to find it. But you can feel that energy with your hands, and you can work with it to help people heal. Zero Balancing is about connecting to this energy in the body, coordinating it with the structure and using that relationship to help create a dynamic stability within the whole system. Through that process we can help healing occur in the body, mind and spirit.

Fritz Smith has a special name for the act of touching both the energy and the structure of the client simultaneously – *donkey touch*. I mentioned this in the last chapter. When we touch the donkey of the person, that is, consciously touch the energy and the structure at the same time, we build an unspoken but strongly felt connection with the client. The donkey represents the animal or instinctual side of us, not our minds and not our logic, but the less linear parts of our selves. We can think of the donkey as parts of us that are not fully under our control – almost

Energy Model

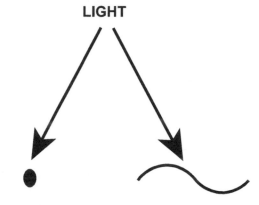

The physics of light

LIGHT

PARTICLE	WAVE
Skeleton	Energy
Ligaments	Movement
Structure	Fields
Matter	Vibration
Form	Force
Mass	Patterns
Texture	Tension
Organization	Abstraction
	Emotion
	Spirit

What can be seen

Tangible
Palpable
Physical
Concrete

What can be experienced

Thoughts
Ideas
Concepts
Belief systems
Childhood strategies
(which did or didn't work out well)
Information
Communication
Consciousness

Fig. 2.1

In Zero Balancing we use light as our model for understanding energy and structure.

(Illustrations by Fritz Smith, used with permission of the Zero Balancing Touch Foundation.)

like our unconscious. In this analogy, the *rider* of the donkey represents the mind. In Zero Balancing, when the client is met at the levels of both structure and energy, we call this donkey touch. In part, the term highlights the way the client responds from her instinctual self, and not from mind or thought.

There are two metaphors – the sailboat and the sweet spot – that help to elucidate this idea. Fritz loves to use the metaphor of a sailboat. The physical part of the boat (the hull, the mast, the sail, the rudder) represents the structure, and the wind that fills the sail is the energy. By adjusting the relationship between the wind and the sail (i.e., between the energy and the structure of the boat) you can adjust how fast the boat moves and control the direction and efficiency of motion. In Zero Balancing we do the same thing. By adjusting the relationship between the energy and the structure in the body, we can affect the health, the mood and the liveliness of the person. The question then becomes, where does the wind meet the sail in the human body? In Zero Balancing, we work with the bones and the joints as the strongest places to access structure and energy.

The second metaphor is the idea of the *sweet spot*. A tennis racquet is a good tool for this metaphor. If you hit the ball on the wooden edge of the racquet (the structure only) you not only get a terrible shot but it also feels terrible. A shock or a shiver goes through your whole body. If you hit the ball in the center of the racquet, in the sweet spot, the ball not only goes straight to where you aimed, it also goes out faster than it came in, and, in addition, you feel this wonderful vibration. Your whole body lights up. The same thing is true for golf or baseball or any activity with a sweet spot.

In ZB we find those sweet spots particularly in the bones. If we can work at that spot, we not only balance many aspects of the physical structure and alignment, we also help the client connect to his deepest core self, to feel the liveliness and even the bliss of this connection. A client recently said to me that Zero Balancing gave him "access to special new experiences" and helped him be his true self.

Touching the energy and structure of the client has several effects. First, the person feels deeply met, which creates trust. Second, donkey touch

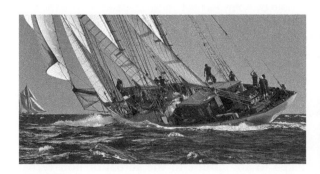

Fig. 2.2
Sailboat – the Boat is the structure and the Wind is the energy.

(Photo: Shutterstock.)

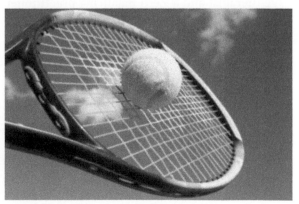

Fig. 2.3
Sweet spot in a tennis racquet.

(Photo: Shutterstock.)

will often move the client into an altered state of consciousness. In that state he is less aware of the external world and more aware of her own internal experience. She is less attached to her normal waking consciousness, less attached to her rigid belief systems and, therefore, more open to change. Some of our erroneous beliefs about ourselves and others ("I am stupid," "I am not good enough," "People don't like me") can shift more easily when we are in this state.

With donkey touch the client moves from the world of duality to the world of unity. Our normal waking consciousness can be described as a world of duality, or as the Chinese put it, *the world of the ten thousand things*. When the client is in the world of unity, he has the experience that there is no time or no space. He feels at one with the environment. This is a deeply meditative state. People often come off the table feeling something major has changed. Sometimes they have a hard time saying what it was. But like Ella in the earlier session, they feel in contact with their true selves in ways they haven't felt "for decades."

Felice is a woman in her thirties who is a massage therapist and a Zero Balancing practitioner. This session was during a ZB class. I asked her to lie on the table so I could show the class how to work on the upper ribs in the back. With Felice lying on her back, I slid my hands underneath her body down to about the eighth thoracic ribs on both sides. There was a lot of held tension in the muscles, but I wanted to feel beneath the muscles down to the structure of the ribs themselves. As I did that, I felt areas of tension in the ribs, like a knot in a tree limb. These were areas with more density than the rest.

As usual in ZB, I held pressure with my fingers into those areas in the ribs. Usually this will allow change to happen to the rib and often throughout

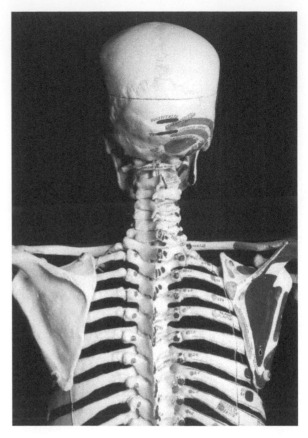

Fig. 2.4

Rib cage and bones of the upper body.

(Photo by Kathy Plunket Versluys. Used with permission of the Zero Balancing Touch Foundation.)

the body. The problem in this session was the ribs were unyielding. The structure of the bones was not shifting at all. The physical structure clearly needed work but some part of her was not willing to let this happen. The practitioner can listen to the messages from the bones in the same way you listen to and attune to the verbal or non-verbal messages of a person. The bones tell you what they want, if you can hear, in the same way a potter can feel the texture of the clay and know what needs to happen to it.

As I tuned in to the energetic sensations, it felt as if I didn't even have permission to be there. The donkey was saying it wasn't going to move and that the ribs weren't ready for me to have my fingers there and certainly not ready to change. I almost felt pushed away.

So I got a clear message from the ribs, and the donkey, that they were not ready to move. They were not trusting me, or not trusting my hands. The density and hardness was not shifting. My solution to this situation was to stop trying to do anything and to stay connected with the tension without trying to change it. I waited with a neutral attitude and listened to see if movement would begin, or if the donkey would give me permission to help.

It took a long time. I just stayed present, listening to what I felt in my hands and in her bones. I listened to the donkey, to the energy and to the structure of the ribs. I didn't move away physically and I didn't leave energetically. I was right there with light pressure even though she wasn't sure she wanted me there. I waited at least a minute or two.

Finally, I felt movement begin. I finally felt invited in. I felt enough trust on the part of the tissues that change could start and the client could begin to let things move and free up. I felt the tension begin to lessen. When that happened the ribs changed a lot. They became more relaxed, softer and more lively and vibrant. It felt good to me and to her. As the tension in her structure let go, she had numerous deep breaths and could relax much more. The benefit of waiting for the donkey to be present was big in this case.

This made me feel we had established a good rapport between Felice's donkey and me. Or said another way, we had made a connection between Felice and her unconscious. I thought that this quality of connection would remain constant after

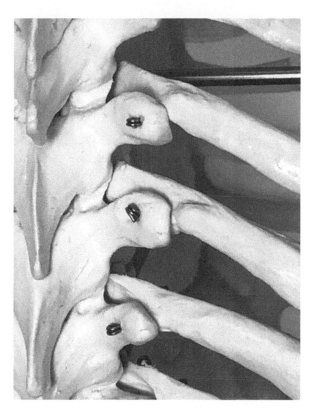

Fig. 2.5

Each rib articulates with the spine in three places – one with the transverse process of one vertebra and also with the body of that vertebra and the vertebra above. So fulcrums placed on a rib affect that rib, the connected vertebrae, the ligaments that hold these articulations together and the effect is then transmitted to the rest of the spine and the skeleton.

(Photo: James McCormick.)

that, and all the rest of the session would come easily. But when I went to the next rib higher up in the body, the same thing happened all over again. It was as if that rib had no communication with the previous rib or no knowledge of the experience that rib had just had. We were right back to the rib not moving, either structurally or energetically, and the donkey not being willing to let go.

So again I stayed present, listening and waiting to feel the energy. I waited for the donkey to let me know that I could work. Again there was at least a minute or more of waiting until the message came through to me, "I am okay now. You can work." I felt the energy in the tissue suddenly soften and yield. There was movement where before there had been none. There was liveliness in the tissues that hadn't been there before. The donkey has a consciousness and can communicate this way if we listen.

I went deeper with the fulcrum into her ribs, and the energy in the bone began to shift even more. What had felt hard and resistant and unmoving kept moving. The tissue got lighter, softer and more flexible. The knot in the bone began to disappear. This was accompanied by deep breaths and deep relaxation by Felice, and felt really good to her. Now I was sure I would be able to go ahead and work, and the donkey would have enough trust and safety to let the work happen. After all, I had just spent a lot of time getting connected, building trust and proving my constancy. Surely these two experiences had been felt by all of Felice, including her donkey and her unconscious.

In ZB we check all of the ribs and work on those that need attention, so I moved on to the next higher rib. Much to my surprise we went through the exact same experience again. This rib had the same resistant and unmoving quality and required just as much time and listening and waiting as the others. Yet with patient connecting, it eventually moved. The same thing happened with the fourth rib.

Only after working on four or five ribs, all of which had a positive outcome once the connection was made, did these experiences translate to the body as a whole. From then on the whole system was much more trusting, accessible and able to move. The donkey was present, and both the structure and the energy body were responding.

Talking afterwards, Felice felt very positive about the experience, especially my willingness to wait and be present. She agreed that it was true she had been resistant, and also that it was true she needed that degree of safety and presence for that length of time in order to feel safe. It took that quality of connection for her to feel I wasn't going to abandon her.

The next thing Felice said after the session was, "Where were you?" She said it angrily, as if asking why hadn't I been there much earlier in her life. Her tone seemed to ask why had I abandoned her, as if I had been the one who was not present in her childhood. We didn't discuss who this really referred to, but this feeling was definitely from way back in her life and about someone in her family. Her feelings of having been abandoned (physically and emotionally) had translated into not feeling safe, not feeling met, and thus not willing to meet others. She was unable to trust that the other would stay present. This had literally translated into her body where her ribs were held tightly, both the structure and the energy. They were not going to change their stance without sufficient proof of constancy and presence over time.

This ended up being a major session for Felice, letting her see how she had protected herself in a way that had been necessary at one time, but had since become almost a prison of isolation, keeping her from connecting to others. Helping to make this shift in her body helped her to make the same shift in her life. As she was able to lessen her defensive patterns, she began to feel more at home in her body and to have access to her deeper self.

If we had just worked with the structure, that is, if we had just tuned in to the tension in her bones, and not the energy, it would have helped her also. She would have felt more relaxed. Her ribs would have been somewhat less tight. She would have felt somewhat better. But she would not have had the major experience she had of shifting some of her longest held patterns, a shift that allowed her life going forward to be different.

A ZB session with Charley is another example of the difference between working with just the structure of the person and working with both the energy and the structure. Charley is a psychiatrist in his fifties who loves Zero Balancing and has had numerous sessions. When he came in on this day, his chief complaint was that his right wrist and thumb were sore from target shooting practice at a gun range, which he was doing because it helps his balance. He also has major scoliosis, which is prominent on the right side of his back and distorts his spinal alignment.

While Charley was sitting up, I did a lot of ZB work on his thumb, the carpal bones in the hand, his wrist, forearm, elbow and shoulder. The focus here was more on the structure than the energy and worked with the alignment of the whole arm and hand. The work was extremely helpful. The pain in his wrist and thumb was reduced, and he felt release and relaxation in those areas.

Then Charley lay down, and we did a full Zero Balancing session with more emphasis on the relationship between his structure and his energy. He was very tight on his right lower ribs, where the scoliosis is most prominent. I worked deeply there, deeper than I usually do. I was aiming to get more energetic change in this session to give him more of an experience of the expansive side of ZB, not only the physical effects.

As we worked, Charley's body relaxed and he had many strong working signs. I spent a lot of effort and time connecting to and listening to his structure and energy. I was listening for what he (and his donkey) was asking for and how could I meet his need. He kept letting go more fully, and gradually let himself drop into a place of deep inner awareness. He had long deep breaths, and I felt strong vibrations in his tissues, signs of bigger and deeper change. I held him there as long as possible to extend his time in the experience, which is usually pleasant and was in this case, as well.

At the top of the table, I held his head for a long time without doing anything except paying careful attention to the bones of the skull and the energy in the skull with non-judgment and caring. I just listened, and he continued to drop deeper and deeper. This opening allowed me to work directly on the vertebrae, which is less common in ZB. He went into a place of deep stillness, one form of an altered state of consciousness. Later he said that he had the thought, "Still waters run deep."

He felt great after the session. His eyes looked very bright. He came out of the session talking in a different way. He felt more connected to life and to deeper meaning in his life, and he began to speak about this. We had a long conversation about the effects of bringing two separate things into relationship. In ZB terms, we had brought his energy and his structure into relationship in a way that helped him have an expanded awareness of unity.

We continued to talk for quite a while afterward. He mentioned that in dialectical materialism there is the idea that you bring two contrasting ideas together and they affect each other in such a way that a third new idea merges. In meditation, if you bring two contrasting sensations together at the same time you can go into an altered state.

Yin and *yang* are, of course, two sides of the same coin, as are structure and energy.

In yin/yang theory, the proportions of yin and yang vary in every situation with different effects, and we can do the same with structure and energy. When yin and yang are held in the right balance, a new movement is generated. The Chinese say that humans are the product of the relationship between Heaven and Earth, the yin and yang of creation.

In ZB, the relationship between structure and energy held at the same time creates a sense of oneness, a feeling of unity. At one point during the session, Charley said, "When I am shooting I don't think. I pay attention to the gunsight not the target. I may not even see the target. I am paying more attention to my bodily experience and thus to my donkey." I responded, "When I play golf I need to relax the body and feel the club head. I need not to be thinking too much. I need not to be living in *the rider*."

"The way I do psychiatry," he responded, "is to listen so carefully that the client and I become one, and then we may not even need words. And to do that I also need to pay full attention to my own voice and my own heart."

Charley kept sharing more about how he was feeling and what he wanted in life. "All of life is about getting to that place of just being – with joy and nothing to do. And I am in that place – that core place where we become ZERO. Zero is nothing but also everything. I want to get to a place of relaxed attention where I don't think. It's really non-doing." To me this was gratifying, and it also gave evidence of the effect of bringing the energy and structure of the person into a balanced relationship and letting the body take over from there.

A last note on donkeys: in Zero Balancing we often say we want donkey-on-donkey touch. That is, we want to touch the clients' donkey and also to reach out from our own donkey. We want the Zero Balancer to be in her instinctual self, as well as the client. Working from our structure and energy to the client's structure and energy creates the deepest kind of connection and allows even more to happen in the session. As the Zero Balancer feels more connected to her core self, she can move into a state of unity as well, which allows the client to expand even further.

Chapter 3
Foundation Joints

In the last chapter we talked about energy and structure, particle and wave and the way in which the wind meeting the sail is the perfect metaphor for energy meeting structure. The next question is, where does this happen in the body? Where does the wind meet the sail in the body? Where can we most influence the relationship between energy and structure?

In ZB, there are two answers: First, in the bones. We will see in Chapter 4 how the bones carry a deep part of our energetic capacity. They are a place in Zero Balancing where we can strongly influence the relationship between energy and structure. The other main place where we can most strongly affect energy and structure is at the joints and, in particular, a group of joints known as the *foundation joints*.

Foundation joints

Foundation joints have several defining characteristics:

1. **They have a minute range of motion.** An example of foundation joints is the set of the cranial bones in the skull. Among bodyworkers, there is some discussion of whether there is movement at all in these bones, but our view is that there is minute movement, in the range of six microns – that is, six one-thousandths of an inch. Extremely small. Compare that to the amount of movement you have in your shoulder joint or your hip joint, which are not foundation joints. The list of foundation joints (and semi-foundation joints) includes the articulation between the cranial bones of the skull; joints between the vertebrae and the between the ribs and the vertebrae; the joint where the sternum meets the manubrium in the chest; the sacroiliac joint in the pelvis; the carpal bones in the hand and the tarsal bones in the feet.

2. **There is no voluntary musculature across these joints.** There is no voluntary muscle that allows you to move one vertebrae in your back just by itself. You can move that vertebrae but only by moving your whole spine, similar to the parietal bone

on the side of your skull. You cannot move that bone just by itself. You can move your whole head, but not just that one bone.

3. **Because there are no voluntary muscles across these joints, problems that arise there tend to stay there.** If you develop soreness or restriction in your elbow, for instance, you can move it around, and there are numerous things you do to help heal it. But problems in the foundation joints can't be easily addressed, and thus tend to last longer. They are often beneath the conscious awareness of the person, another reason they don't get addressed.

4. This point is very important. **Because these joints have such a small range of motion, a very small disturbance in their balance makes for a huge loss of function.** If the range of motion of a joint is 6 microns, if they lose 3 microns of motion they have lost 50% of their range and 50% of their function. The corollary to this is that a very small improvement in these joints will lead to a very large improvement of function. This is one of the reasons that Zero Balancing is not about how hard or how deep the touch is. We only need to make small changes in these key areas to make a large improvement for the person.

5. Lastly, and most important of all, what is the function we are talking about? If a joint loses 50% of

its function, what exactly is the function that is being lost? With our main joints, those that are not foundation joints, like ankles or knees or hips, the first function that gets lost is locomotion. But that is not the case with these small foundation joints. **One of the key insights from Zero Balancing is that the main function of these foundation joints is the transmission of energetic forces through the body.** For instance, the tarsal bones in the feet below the ankle joint are all foundation joints (the joints between the calcaneus, the talus, the cuboid and the cuneiforms). If these joints get compromised, what is lost is the energetic transmission through these bones – in this case leading to a lack of connection between the feet and the ground. The person will literally feel less grounded and less supported. Similarly, if the cranial bones are not functioning properly you will lose the connection between your skull and the heavens.

So these joints are crucial to the energetic functioning of the body. When any of these joints is compromised, we tend to lose awareness of and connection to that part of our bodies – usually without being aware of it. We are less in touch with our whole self. We are getting less information from that part of our selves. This can sometimes have small effects and sometimes quite large effects. With Zero Balancing we can evaluate the functioning of all of the crucial foundation joints and balance them as needed, thus helping many

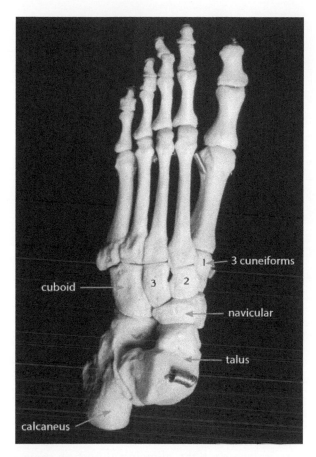

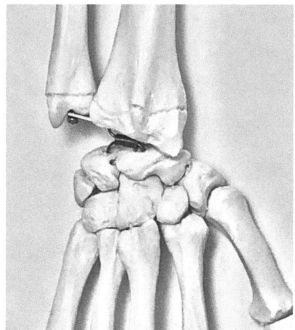

Fig. 3.1

All the articulations between the bones named in this photo are true foundation joints, with very small range of motion and no voluntary muscles across them.

(Photo by Kathy Plunket Versluys. Used with permission of the Zero Balancing Touch Foundation.)

Fig. 3.2

Carpal bones of the hand. All the articulations between these bones are also true foundation joints.

(Photo: James McCormick.)

physical issues, but also helping the person feel more connected to himself.

A few case studies can show the power of working with the foundation joints.

Work with a client early in my ZB practice showed me the importance of the foundation joints in significant physical injuries. Rose was rear-ended in a major car accident one year in September. She had a lot of pain after the accident, focusing in her right sacroiliac joint (the major foundation joint in the pelvis in the lower back). She also had significant pain in both her left and right hip and in her neck.

She came in for Zero Balancing eleven days after the accident. During the preceding eleven days the pain had continued and had become worse. When I evaluated her, the main finding was extremely limited motion in the foundation joint on the right side of her lower back at the sacroiliac joint. The tissue and the energy there

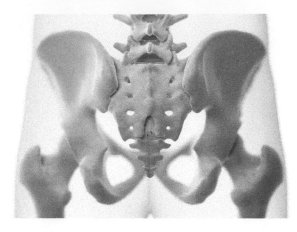

Fig. 3.3

Pelvis showing the sacrum and the sacro-iliac joint.

(Photo: Shutterstock.)

felt hard and rigid. Even though there was pain in several other places, the SI joint was the most limited area from the accident, so during the Zero Balancing session I focused mostly on the energetic disturbance there.

After the first session, all of the pains, not just her back, were 50% better. Her motion at the joint was much improved and the energy in the joint felt softer, with more flow. I saw her one more time a week later. My findings were similar. The strongest imbalance was still in the foundation joint at the right SI joint, but it was much less imbalanced. The motion had held its improvement and the energy present in the joint was also clearer and stronger.

Due to a combination of circumstances, I didn't see her again until a month later. At that time, she was 90% better after the two sessions and had maintained that improvement. She felt very little pain, and my findings matched hers, with nearly normal function in the joint. She was also much better in her hips and neck, as well as her back.

I learned several things from my work with Rose. First, I learned how quickly the changes can come from focusing on these joints. Second, these sessions reinforced the idea that balancing the foundation joints allows the transmission of energetic forces throughout the whole body, not just the local area. In this case, freeing up the SI joint had released energy that had been held there, and created a clearer, stronger field of energy in her whole system.

Ernie is a man is his forties from California. He came in for some Zero Balancing sessions and began to talk about his life. He said he had very good skills in his field, but was unrecognized and unknown, which was frustrating to him. He was hoping that Zero Balancing could help him in some way. I was unsure but agreed to evaluate and see what I could find. In this case I decided to evaluate all the foundation joints in his body before the session, to see if I could find any major imbalances that might relate to what he was saying.

As I did the evaluations, the major discovery was a significant restriction in the tarsal bones in his feet. The ligaments holding the bones together were extremely tight, allowing almost no movement between these joints. The bones themselves felt vague, with low energy, not well defined.

One of our theories in Zero Balancing is that when experiences are not able to be fully processed by our consciousness, that unprocessed information gets stored somewhere in the body as tension or other forms of held energy. We often see the strongest and deepest hurts showing up as held vibration in the bones and in the ligaments joining the bones. In particular, the unprocessed part of our early childhood experience can strongly affect the quality and the movement of the tarsal bones in our feet.

Most children learn to walk between around 10 months and 15 months. As they are first walking, the energetic vibrations in their home and family affect their young systems tremendously and can get reflected in the quality of the vibration in the bones and joints in their feet. The practitioner can literally feel the effects of the client's early life by listening to the quality of the energy in the bones and joints in the tarsal area.

In Ernie's case, once I found strong holding in his tarsal bones and joints, I asked him what his childhood had been like. He told me that he had lived in an environment where children were not supposed to be seen or heard. He had literally learned how to be invisible to his parents by walking and tiptoeing quietly without attracting any attention to himself. This had turned into that same behavior in his adult life, where he was not getting seen or heard or appreciated for his work.

We did several Zero Balancing sessions, working on his whole body, but with particular attention to his feet. Over several sessions, the ligaments in the foundation joints became much more fluid and loose. The bones got more resilient and lively. His walking was easier and he felt much better in himself.

What was most remarkable was that over the next six months he began to receive more notice and acclaim for his work. He was no longer invisible. Our conclusion was that freeing up the old pattern of invisibility stored in the foundation joints in his feet had let him behave differently in his current life, leading to different results.

Mike is a musician in his fifties. He came to see me over the years for both acupuncture and Zero Balancing. The most interesting feature of his Zero Balancing sessions took place in the carpal bones of his hands and happened almost every time I worked on him with ZB. The carpal bones are eight small bones just distal to the wrist joint. They are true foundation joints with all the

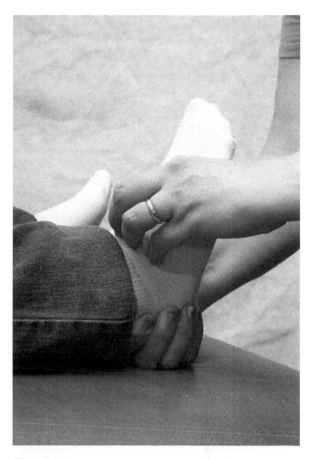

Fig. 3.4

One handed half moon vector to balance the tarsal bones in the foot.

(Photo: Della Watters; WattersWorks & Company.)

characteristics listed above. The carpal bones are the scaphoid, lunate, triquetrum trapezium, trapezoid, hamate, capitate and pisiform.

The session would usually go very well. We would start with the lower half of the body and then work with the upper half. In a typical session there is some Zero Balancing work on the arms in the second half of the session. Mike used his arms a lot in his playing, so I would always give them attention. Each time I would gradually work down his arms until I reached his wrist and hand. As soon as I started to work with the carpal bones in his hands, the whole tenor of the session would change. He would immediately begin to have very deep breaths, followed by a reddening of his face, followed almost immediately by hearty laughter. The energetic feeling in his whole body would change. He would become more relaxed, more energized and livelier. In addition, his mood and voice tone would change dramatically. He would want to, and often did, start to tell jokes and become quite funny. We would both end up laughing about the change with seemingly little work on his hands.

The work on the foundation joints in his hands at the articulation of the carpal bones produced a significantly different response than at any other part of his body. My conjecture was that due to the strain of many years of playing, often in stressful situations, a lot of energetic holding had been created in the carpal bones. As soon as we released some of that holding, we allowed the body to make a connection that had been blocked before. It was like releasing the water behind a dam or re-setting the circuit breaker. Once the connection was made, his whole system responded strongly and positively.

Chapter 4
The Bones Store Our Essence

One of the vital principles of Zero Balancing, and one that sets it apart from most bodywork styles, is our emphasis on working directly with the energy and structure of the skeletal system. Clinically there is a different feeling for both the practitioner and the client when the practitioner is working with the bones rather than the soft tissues (muscles, tendons, fascia). In his book *Inner Bridges*, Dr Smith compares the feeling of working with the energy of the soft tissue to the feeling you experience walking in an apple orchard. The feeling is soft, earthy, horizontal, and very much about the Ten Thousand Things and the earthly realm. In contrast, he describes the feeling of working with the energy of the bones as more like the feeling you get when you walk into a cathedral, ethereal, heavenly and vertical.

Physically, the bones are among the largest, the deepest and the densest tissues in the body, so they carry the strongest and largest currents of energy.

In the ZB model, we believe energy from the universe comes into the body directly through the top of the skull. This is our highest point and functions like a lightning rod. Our view is that this energy infuses all the tissues of the body, but the bones carry the strongest part of this energetic flow. So we can access this universal life force most directly in the bones.

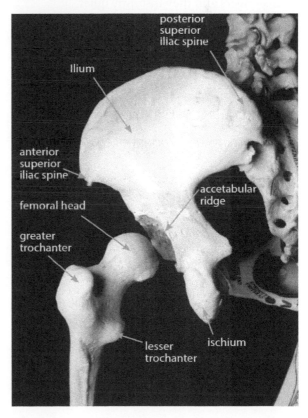

Fig. 4.1

The bones of the pelvis and hip joint.

(Photo: by Kathy Plunket Versluys. Used with permission of the Zero Balancing Touch Foundation.)

21

The Chinese linked the bones to the kidney meridians in acupuncture, and they saw the kidneys' main function as storing the *essence* of our body. This is in keeping with the ZB idea that the bones contain information about a deep part of our being. The bones are ideal for working with energy because bones tend to transmit energy rather than absorb it. A fulcrum into one bone will affect the vibration in the whole skeleton.

Soft tissue, on the other hand, tends to absorb energy. If a drummer wants to stop the sound of the cymbals he touches them with the soft tissue of his fingers and they instantly quiet.

Bones are always changing. We think of them as hard like wood or metal but they are alive, and the body is always adding boney tissue or removing boney tissue. When the astronauts first went into space for extended time they lost 1%–2% of their boney tissue each month. In a weightless environment bones are less needed and they start to get absorbed by the body.

A Zero Balancer will evaluate a bone by feeling its quality and its vitality. Some bones feel more brittle, some more dense or full and some more vibrant and healthy. When we feel areas of particular density or tension in a bone we call it *bone gold*, because we know there is a richness of energy and information stored in that tension. When the energy held there can be freed up, the energy and the information becomes more accessible and more useful to the person.

In bodywork, we will work with a tense part of a client's body, and as the tension releases a strong memory or feeling may arise. These memories arise because at some time in the past a strong experience occurred that the client was not able to accept or process. Some of the emotions around the event are denied or repressed and that leaves an imprint in the body. In Zero Balancing we think (based on our clinical experience) that many of these deepest imprints leave their marks on the bones in the form of irregularities or imbalances.

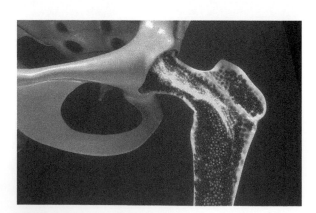

Fig. 4.2

Energy moving through the bones of pelvis and hip.

(Photo: Shutterstock.)

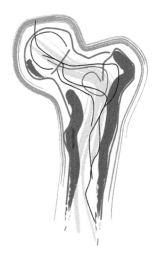

Fig. 4.3

Energy flowing through a bone.

(Credit: Mary Murphy, with permission.)

With Zero Balancing we work to free up those areas of tension or imbalance. As we put a fulcrum, with pressure or traction, into a bone and hold it for as few as 3–10 seconds, not only can we feel the tense place ease, but the whole bone can change its quality. The brittle bone can get less brittle, the dense bone less dense and the bone that is too soft can firm up. The client will then have a corresponding experience. For example, as the dense bone gets less dense, the person will start to feel lighter. Figure 4.4 gives a graphic representation of that process in Zero Balancing.

What's even more amazing and interesting is that, as in the preface with Doug, I can start to feel the quality of the energetic vibration held in a bone. I can feel the signature of an emotion. Anger will feel different from sadness. Indecision can feel different from grief. The practitioner can feel the quality of the held energy, which allows her to tailor the touch to the need of the client. When we work on bony tissue, we are affecting a deep part of the person and working in a way that will allow greater and more fundamental change.

I did a ZB session on Tracy, a woman in her mid-forties, who was an acupuncture student. I performed a full Zero Balancing session on her in front of the acupuncture class. Her main complaints were extreme tightness in her neck and upper back. She also said she had major tension throughout her body. I asked if there was anything else and she said there was some difficulty in her relationship but she did not say more about that.

This was an interesting session right from the start. The very first thing I often do in a session when the client is lying down is put my hands gently on the bones in her shins (the tibia). This has several purposes. One is to say hello to the person with my hands and to allow us to connect and begin to feel comfortable with each other.

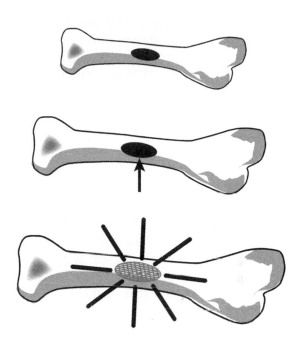

Fig. 4.4

The dark circle in the bone represents bone held energy ("bone gold") where an energetic disturbance has caused an area of density or dysfunction in the bone, which can be perceived by the Zero Balancer. When the ZBer places a fulcrum into the bone where the energy is held (on a rib this would be a simple fulcrum lifting towards the ceiling) as shown in the second picture, that held energy is dispersed, allowing that holding pattern to let go and allowing the energy to return to the general circulation where it can be more available to the person. This tends to feel very good, gives the receiver the experience of more energy and allows some deep-seated disturbance to heal.

(Credit: James McCormick.)

The other is to assess the state of the energy in the bones. The shin bones are prominent and covered only by a thin layer of skin and tissue, so it is an easy place to make direct contact with the bones.

The sensation I felt in Tracy's tibias was remarkable, quite different from what I commonly feel. The assessment was clear, like reading someone's pulse in Chinese medicine. The energetic sensation was of too much hardness and density. They felt not only hard but also tight. This was especially striking and unexpected to me since she was a slight, thin woman. There was also a lot of fluid in the tissues, and the result was a feeling of rigidity in her whole leg as well as the tension in the shin. I immediately mentioned to the class what I had felt and how striking it was.

The work on Tracy's lower body was of high quality, and she experienced a lot of energetic change as we worked on the bones of her lower ribs, her pelvis, her hips and her feet. She felt more and more relaxed as we went along, and she kept saying over and over how good it all felt and how surprised she was. She was having many working signs of energetic change, including rapid eyelid flutter, deep breaths and borborygmus. I felt the hardness and tension in her bones gradually relaxing.

Halfway through the session, at the end of the work on her lower body, I re-checked the shin bones to see how they felt. This is one way of monitoring the amount of change in the session and the quality of the change. Her bones were much lighter, freer and softer. I mentioned to the class what I was feeling, to which she responded, "I feel very much lighter, especially in my legs. I feel like floating." This was a dramatic change in her from before the session, and we were only halfway through. The bones literally change their quality. In Figure 4.4 you can see another metaphorical image for how the bone shifts with ZB fulcrums

and how that allows greater transmission of energy through the bone and through the whole system.

We continued the session, working with the upper ribcage, the cervical vertebrae, and the skull. By the end of the full session her bones felt totally different. They felt light, not heavy or dense. The bones had much more flow and liveliness. More importantly, she felt the same way. She felt "a great deal of change. My legs feel so light I feel like floating. I feel totally happy and relieved." She had a lot less tension both in her body and in her being. "I feel like a weight has been lifted." She felt wonderful and grateful. It was good to see how the change in the bones, and in her body, mirrored the change in her mood and sense of self.

Watching her as she lay on the table after the session, it was easy to see that energy was flowing in her whole body. She was relaxed, and I could see the sparkle in her eyes and the depth and ease of her breathing. She had much more vitality. She felt her "whole body connected," and she felt "back to my real self," which is a phrase we hear over and over again after a ZB session.

Tracy lay on the table for a while after I finished working. She was still feeling good and grateful. And then, in a moment, she suddenly started to get sad and cry. This was surprising and embarrassing to her. She didn't understand why she was suddenly so sad when she had been feeling so happy. To me this was common and no cause at all for concern. In fact, it is one more sign of a significant experience.

When someone has a major change from a session they often feel great immediately afterward and then get sad. There can be many reasons. Sometimes people feel embarrassed, as if they have revealed too much of themselves or revealed a weakness. This can be especially true in a group setting.

When this is the case, I reassure the person in great detail and depth that what they have just done is wonderful. It takes courage to share so much of yourself. It takes courage to feel your feelings to that degree. So I support and acknowledge the person for her courage and the work she has done.

Other times there is a phenomena called *mourning of the self*, which we saw earlier with Ella in the preface. People start to get sad when they see how much they have missed by having these static patterns that didn't allow them to move or fully live. They realize they could have been having this wonderful feeling years ago, and they feel sad for themselves. They now have enough courage, freedom and support to tolerate and deal with strong feelings, when formerly they didn't.

There are so many things to learn from this session, but in terms of the significance of working with the bones there are some clear highlights. Much of the person's state, both emotional and physical, is readable through paying attention to the quality of the energy in the bones. The tightness I felt in Tracy's bones mirrored exactly what she felt in her body and in her being, both before, during and after the session.

Touching the bones and listening to their messages helps make a connection to a deep part of the person. Working directly with the bones through traction, compression or torque can make a huge shift in the quality of the bones and the quality of the person's experience. Also, I can monitor the change in the person by monitoring the change in the bones, as the bones are a good reflection of what is happening overall for the person.

A session with Helen, a long-time client in her forties, is another example of how working with the bones has a deep effect on the person. This

session was in January. Helen's mother had died the previous year. She felt a great deal of grief and disruption to her life while going through that experience. This was a difficult period for her, as only she and her brother remained in the family.

Then, without warning, she heard from her brother that his daughter, who was young, lovely and lively, fell off her bicycle and died from the fall. She had been in good health. There was total shock and devastation for everyone, friends and family. Helen and her husband went to the funeral and comforted her brother and the family as best they could.

This was the first time I had seen her since she heard the news. She came in saying she was feeling "weird, disconnected, feeling a lot of grief and fear and feeling very vulnerable." When I saw her walk in the door I thought she was in shock. She looked disoriented. She seemed almost outside of herself and not present in her body.

The frame for the session was difficult to find. Helen wasn't sure what she wanted or needed. She talked in a rambling way for a while and finally said, "I feel I have a hole in my heart." She started crying and said, "I just want to feel carefree. I just want to be happy. Things are always so hard. I feel like I am just kind of slogging through. I am getting through one day at a time. When do I just get to be carefree? I want to feel more fully myself."

We eventually decided this would become the goal, or *frame*, for today's session. We would work to help her deal with her grief, feel more fully herself and more carefree. When we went to the table, the first thing I did was feel her shin bones. They were the opposite of Tracy's shins. They were almost devoid of energy. They felt as if there was nobody home. The technical word for it is *dissociated*, which people use for the mental state of someone in trauma, when her awareness leaves the body. That mental state has a similar effect in the physical body. The tissues, in this case the tibias, lacked vitality. They had a very low charge and a very low presence. When I asked Helen what she felt in those bones, she said, "They are kind of empty and they need to be filled up." As her description perfectly matched the sensation I was feeling, I knew I was on the right path.

I like to understand ideas through metaphors. A very good metaphor for a person with a dissociation of energy is the taste and feeling of a tomato in January, at least in the Northeast. Tomatoes at that time are often hard and have little Ch'i and little taste. They have the consistency of cardboard. Compare that to a tomato in August, which feels so lively and is so juicy and tasty you can have a dinner with just the tomato and some mozzarella and basil. That tomato has Ch'i. The bones of a healthy, vibrant person feel like the tomato in August. The bones of someone who is dissociated feel empty. That was the case with Helen's shin bones that day.

I started the work on her lower body, but quickly went to her upper body. This was outside our normal protocol, but I felt she really needed connection there. I immediately felt the hardness in her ribs. As we went on she said, "I feel the effect in my chest. I can feel the hole in my heart." I asked her to tolerate feeling that hole in her heart without trying to change it. I continued to hold my connection to bones in her rib cage, and I asked her to be curious and friendly to what she felt, to invite it in rather than push it away. This work is based on techniques developed many years ago by Chicago-based psychologist Eugene Gendlin, a technique he called *focusing*. She was able to stay with this feeling in her body, but she felt very "vulnerable." She felt a "fear of this happening to others, of others dying. I don't know if I can do this again. I don't want to spend all my time wondering when the next person is going to die."

Being able to stay with the sensations in her chest allowed those sensations of fear and vulnerability to begin to change. Gradually she began to feel the hole in her heart grow smaller and be somewhat less painful. I worked lightly, but with a lot of connection. I paid attention to her rib cage, both posteriorly and anteriorly. I also did a lot of ZB on the bones in her chest, her sternum and her manubrium. If I found a place where the energy moved a lot, and which felt really good to her, I stayed longer and let that build. Like the shins, these bones had started out empty and without much Ch'i. As we worked there, and as she continued to let herself feel what was happening in her chest, the bones began to change as well, becoming more full and lively.

I held the bones of Helen's skull a long time at one point, without doing much pressure or movement. I was being present, compassionate and caring, and working to communicate that through my touch. She still had a lot of sad and difficult feelings, but she also began to feel much more alive and present and able to cope.

I finished the session on her lower body and did a long fulcrum of compassion on her feet. At the end, she asked me to go back and work with her arms, which I did, and this felt really good to her. At the end of the session I assessed the quality of her shin bones. They no longer felt empty. They were filled with vitality. Helen was inhabiting her bones and her body. She no longer felt the hole in her heart. She felt much better – softer, lighter, less worried and more connected to herself. This had been her goal at the beginning. She felt much more able to cope with the difficult events in her life and in her family. And she felt grateful. The Zero Balancing session, especially the work on her bones, had made a big change in her body but even more so on her well-being.

Chapter 5
Living in the Moment

Another essential aspect of Zero Balancing is that we touch in a particular way, which we call *interface touch*. This means the Zero Balancer keeps her attention at the place where her hand meets the body of the client. That is, she keeps at least part of her attention at the physical boundary between the practitioner and the person on the table.

There are many benefits to using this kind of touch. For one, the boundary is clear. There is no blurring. There is no sense that the practitioner invades the space of the client, or that the client can invade the space of the Zero Balancer. They feel connected without any fuzziness. It is two responsible, independent adults meeting with no co-dependence going on. Both parties feel safe. The client has the experience of being met in a respectful way. This allows him to relax more and to allow the session to happen in a deeper way.

Also, there is clear communication. The touch is not a barrier. The Zero Balancer can feel a lot of what is happening in the body and mind of the client, through the connection at the interface. Using this style of touch, the ZBer can work with the energy of the client without sending or streaming any of her own energy to the client. If the ZBer wants to help increase the energy of the receiver, she doesn't send her own energy. Instead, she helps to activate the client's energy.

Some students of ZB find this is one of the most important lessons of the class. If they feel a fuzziness or lack of clarity in their connection to the client, they learn that they are unconsciously blending or streaming energy with their touch. They often then realize they are having this same lack of clarity in other parts of their lives as well. They also become aware how this tendency has caused them confusion and left them tired or out of sorts.

I have a friend who is a chiropractor who took a ZB class for the first time around 20 years ago. Afterward, she moved away from the area and I did not see her for a while. I saw her again last year, and she still talks about what a difference learning interface touch made to her practice and to her life. She was able to get much more connected to her clients and thus to work more deeply with less effort. She began to live at interface, where she felt her own feelings, and those of others, without trying to change any of them. This allowed her to become much more present in her life and her work. She felt more focused, more in touch with her core self and more able to be present to others. She thinks this was one of her most important lessons from Zero Balancing.

As she learned about interface touch, she was more able to be conscious of *what is real,* rather than being confused by her projections or wishes. She learned to be more in the moment. All of these are major lessons that go far beyond learning ZB.

At the beginning of my ZB practice I had to concentrate on being at interface all the time. While I was working on someone, I had to think, "Where is my attention? Is my attention on my fingertips where I meet the person?" Whenever I noticed that I wasn't at interface, I would usually notice that I was less in touch with the client. As soon as I brought my attention back to interface in my fingertips, I was automatically back in touch with the client as well. It was a bit like meditating. If I let my mind drift, I was no longer with the client, and the work had to be less effective.

Today, I don't need to pay much conscious attention to interface when I do Zero Balancing. My body has learned to work in that way all the time. It is now my default setting, and I work at interface without thinking about it. This leaves me much more bandwidth to pay attention to the client. I can also give better attention to my own internal body signals, which become more and more important as practitioners get more experience in Zero Balancing.

A ZB session I did with Max is a good example of what happens when the practitioner is out of touch with interface, and it shows what happens when he gets back to interface. Max is a psychologist in his forties who has had a long history of experience with Zero Balancing. Halfway into this session, I wasn't feeling much change in his body, his energy or his emotion. He was talking about his week and all that was happening but

without really expressing much emotion. He had a lot of self-condemnation, guilt and shame, along with a lot of fear and anxiety. But he was talking about these things and thinking about them, not actually feeling the feelings.

The work on the whole of the lower body went along in this way with only small changes. When I arrived at the upper body, the ZB fulcrums to the ribs and the heart area also seemed to make little difference. At this point in the session I realized that I was feeling a lot of guilt (at not helping him to change more) and anxiety (that he would be upset with me for not getting him better). Max was someone who had become a friend over time and was a mental health professional whom I respected, so I wanted him to see me as a "good" practitioner.

I finally realized that as I was working I had most of my awareness on my own thoughts. I was thinking about whether I was doing a good job and what I would say if nothing changed. I wasn't at interface at all. My attention was not on my fingertips or even on him. I was spending too much of my attention worrying about me and feeling anxiety.

As soon as I realized that, I knew immediately what to do. I needed to get back to interface where my hands met Max's body, where he would feel met and I would get the information I needed to help him. I was able to return my attention to my fingertips and just tune in to the sensations I felt there. Rather than worrying about whether things would change, or even trying to change things, being calm at the interface allowed me to get in touch with what was there, without judging it or trying to change it.

I immediately felt the strong tension in his body. The tissue was so tight that very little movement was happening. The strongest sensation I noticed was a significant degree of holding on. Once the information started coming, more insight came with it. I was able to understand that he held things so tightly because he didn't feel worthy. And because he was holding himself so tightly, he was not able to let in love, compassion, help or caring.

I went to Max's head and held his head in my hands for a long time. I tuned in further, at interface, and then said to him, "Let yourself accept the caring and the help. See if you can let go into my help and the compassion and caring I have for you."

Structural Touch

One touches the structure of another person without consciously and knowingly engaging their energy.

Essential Touch

One makes an energetic connection with another person, with or without physical contact. For example, we can "touch" the energy body by listening to a person's voice or by making a connection through sight.

Donkey Touch

One simultaneously and consciously touches both the energy and structure of another person to connect with their core.

Interface Touch

Touching with a clear structural and energetic boundary. Desired mode of touch used that characterizes Zero Balancing, one of its Hallmarks.

Blending Touch

Overlapping of boundaries. There is no clear author of the experience but rather combined vibration of both people. Many other bodywork modalities use blending touch in a beautiful way. In Zero Balancing we use Interface.

Streaming Touch

One sends one's own energy into the client.

Channeling Touch

One becomes a conduit for energy, not its source. This is not to be confused with naturally conducting energy from above down, in that all upright beings (trees, people, etc.) conduct energy.

When we give a Zero Balancing session, we use Donkey Touch at Interface.

Fig. 5.1

Vocabulary of touch – different ways of working with energy. In Zero Balancing we use interface touch.

(Illustrations by Fritz Smith, used with permission of the Zero Balancing Touch Foundation.)

This immediately changed things in the session. His body visibly, physically, let go. He actually moved lower into the table and let a lot of tension go. He started crying, which he did for a full five minutes while also feeling his rage for his father.

This was a big release. Afterward he felt much clearer and less confused. He felt less anxiety (though it was certainly not gone), and his body felt lighter and clearer. A solution to one of the problems he had talked about suddenly appeared without his even thinking about it. His brain was suddenly working more creatively.

My main lesson from this session was to keep my attention on what I was feeling at the interface boundary, and on what was happening in my hands, rather than on my own anxieties or planning. Once I got in touch with Max's donkey, I could let the donkey guide me. His donkey let me know how I could help his energy move. Once we got his energy moving, solutions presented themselves.

There was another interesting session with a client early in my career where I was able to stay at interface the whole time, but the client was not there. I was working with a woman in her forties who was fairly new to Zero Balancing and whom I knew, but not well. The whole first half of the session was difficult for me, as I could not feel anything changing in her body, her energy or her mood. She was very quiet. I was at interface the whole time with my hands, and though I could feel one part of her clearly, that part was not changing at all. This is unusual. I remember thinking to myself, "I better get a new profession because clearly I have no skill at Zero Balancing."

I felt frustrated and couldn't understand why things inside her were not moving.

When I got to the second half of the session, on her upper body, I asked her how she was doing. She mumbled something not very clear, but I thought there was anger in her voice. I asked her if she was angry. It turned out that she was very angry with her father, and I reminded her of her father. Consequently, she had been very angry with me and had been trying not to let anything happen. This is the opposite of interface. She was not present to the moment or to the possibilities of the ZB. She had been in almost complete transference and acting out her anger at her father by not connecting with me. This was mind-blowing at the time, as it was the first time I had encountered this behavior. Her response led to a pause in the ZB session and a long talk, where we got clear that I was not her father, that the time with him was in the past and we were here in the present. We talked about ways in which I was similar to him and ways in which I was different.

Once our conversation was over and we were both clear about our real relationship, the rest of the ZB was excellent. We were both able to stay at interface the rest of the session. I stayed in clear connection with her and she stayed in clear connection with herself, with me and with the present moment. She allowed movement to happen, which resulted in big changes in her tension and anger. Her body felt very different in this part of the session. Our positive connection deepened, and she finished the session feeling wonderful in her body and about herself. Also, her feelings about her father had gotten much clearer by the end.

Chapter 6
Working Signs

There are several ways to notice and monitor the change in the client during a ZB session. The practitioner can often feel the changes in her hands, whether the change happens in the tissues or the energy field or both. Or she might feel a change in her own body, which is responding to something shifting in the client. Sometimes the practitioner can see the change in the energy field, though different practitioners have different experiences of seeing the energy field in a client. Some people see layers of color in the aura.

In addition, the practitioner might also notice physical signs of energy movement that are more easily observable. As I mentioned before, we call these the *working signs*. They are manifestations from the body that the client is in a *working state*. The working state is the period when the client is experiencing and integrating the changes that have been initiated by the Zero Balancing session and often involves an expanded or altered state of consciousness. This often continues even after the session is over.

The working signs can be used by the practitioner to monitor the client's response to the ZB session and to help alter the fulcrums if necessary. There are four major working signs:

> ### Working signs
>
> *The eyes* – If the eyes are open we look for a blank stare, where the eyeballs are not moving and not focused. If we put in a fulcrum on a client and they go into this fixed, blank stare, that means their awareness has gone inside to their experience, and they are no longer paying attention to the outside world. They are having a period of time when their energy and structure are rearranging. This is usually accompanied by a pleasurable feeling and is a reliable sign of significant change.
>
> If the eyes are closed, we look for rapid eyelid flutter or rapid eyeball movement, and these have the same meaning. These are indicators of the person going into an altered state of consciousness – large or small – but less aware of the outside world.

The breath – We look for either a very shallow breath after we put in a fulcrum, or a very deep breath. Either of these is a significant indicator of energetic change, though a prolonged shallow breath may have a different meaning and may be a sign of the person feeling depleted.

The voice – If we are still unsure of how a session is going, we can ask, "How are you?" We are interested in the words the person will say, but much more interested in the tone of the voice. Is it vibrant and lively (a sign of good change)? Or is it a kind of dull monotone (indicative of a depleted field and meaning we need to change the course of the session)?

Slight movements of the head – We look for either a tilting of the head to one side or a tremulous, slightly shaky movement of the head. When I see these signs during a session I know the client is having an energetic experience and her energetic state is shifting inside.

Anne is a woman in her thirties who works at a health care facility. She has received ZB for a number of years, coming pretty regularly. She came in to see me in late December for a ZB session. She said it was a New Year's gift to herself. She came in feeling good, and during the framing process she said she had no particular issues she wanted to address, so we left unspecified what the goal for the session would be. This session with her shows how the working signs can be used to assess the impact a session is having on the client and can also indicate how to adjust the session in response to the working signs.

At the beginning of the session I was having trouble getting connected to her. I was having trouble feeling her energy (feeling her donkey), and it seemed to me that not much was changing within her. She was not showing the working signs. When I asked how she was doing, her voice tone also indicated depletion. It was quiet and lacking vitality.

I wasn't sure why there wasn't much change. When I am not seeing any working signs in the client and I am not feeling a lot of change I start to look to what I can do differently to help the client move. There is a tendency, especially for a beginning Zero Balancer, but for me as well, to think it is my fault. Maybe something I am doing, or not doing, is preventing the energy from moving. In this session I had to keep telling myself, "Don't get discouraged. Don't just go through the motions." And also, "Pay attention and feel what is going on in her even though you don't feel much movement at the moment." I said to myself, "Make room for her donkey."

Still, even with this re-focusing and doing my best to pay attention to the donkey, I was not feeling much happening, and I was still not seeing the working signs I was looking for. I was feeling some frustration. Finally, I heard my inner voice say, "Accept Anne where she is. Just listen. You don't need to try to fix her or change her." And, "Don't judge her or look negatively at her because there isn't much energetic movement."

As I told this to myself, I was able to change my attitude and tune in more to her and less to my worries, similar to the session with Max in Chapter 5. This brought me back to interface with the client. As I began to accept her exactly as she was, and to let go of my need to change her, I began to get more contact and more information, leading me to make three changes in how I was working.

I worked much more slowly. I held the fulcrums longer and took longer pauses between fulcrums. These were all to allow her being to express itself, rather than deal with my input. I wanted to let her donkey and her innate wisdom take over and move the way it wanted to. I got out of the way and just listened to and followed her donkey. I also began to work more lightly and softly.

These changes allowed her physical body and energy body to begin to shift internally and allowed me to feel more connected to her. She felt my connection and thus allowed herself to be seen. We got on an upward spiral. I finally began to see a lot of the working signs. Her breathing changed and she began to have periods of shallow breathing followed by full, deep breaths. Her eyes were closed the whole time, but the eyelids began to have the characteristic flutter of someone whose energy is shifting. Her head began to tilt to the side and to gently, almost imperceptibly, shake. All of these signs told me we were now on the right path.

As Anne's working signs increased, I could feel more energy movement under my hands, and I could literally see waves of motion moving through her body. I had the image of a fish swimming under the surface of the ocean. What I was observing seemed to feel deeply good to her, which she confirmed after the session.

About that time, she said out loud, "I am doing the wave inside, like at a baseball game. I can't stop myself. I've never done that before." The words were so clear and almost matched what I had felt in her body moments earlier, even though I wasn't entirely sure what she meant. Her voice tone as she spoke was wonderful, vibrant, alive and enthusiastic. I asked her "How does that feel?" She said, "It feels wonderful."

I felt totally connected to her donkey and to her at this point. I was able to read how the energy was moving inside, which was confirmed by her words, her voice and her working signs. Now we were surfing together following the wave.

After a few minutes of this surfing, I looked up at Anne's face and expected to see her with a beautiful smile and instead she had a sad face. I was surprised, as she had just been feeling "wonderful," so I asked her, "What are you feeling?" She started to cry and said, "I feel sad but also I feel good. My sister told me I needed a ZB session, and I felt so grateful to her for caring about me."

Once things start to be unblocked in the person, and energy starts to move, many things can happen. Sometimes the person will continue the expansion and just feel better and better. Sometimes she gets frightened because the expansion is new. Sometimes she can just feel touched by the caring of someone and that can bring tears. In this case, Anne got sad but sort of a happy-sad.

As the session went along I kept the fulcrums light with long pauses. I continued to feel more and more connectedness and more and more movement in her. She continued to have even more working signs with even deeper breaths, more rapid eye flutters, whole body relaxation and deep sighs, all the signs of a deeply moving session.

At some point Anne was having such strong signs of energy movement that I asked again, "What is happening now?" Sometimes in ZB the practitioner doesn't talk much to the client during the session, as we want to help a person stay in the right brain and the expanded state of consciousness. Talking may cause a client to think, which may take her out of the feeling state where more powerful change can happen. In this case Anne was able to talk and still stay connected to her deeper self.

She said, "I had this new vision which I've never had before. A vision of a planet that at first I thought was earth. It was golden, a beautiful golden planet, and it made me so happy seeing it. I just observed it. It popped up into my consciousness with no effort on my part. It was something totally new and made me very happy."

Something that is new and has never happened before is significant, and it's a good idea to slow things down and take some time with it. I suggested she let it in and let it affect her. "Let the joy sink into your nervous system and even into your soul, so it gets imprinted there." The more we talked about her vision of a beautiful golden planet, the happier she got. And while there was still sadness as well, she was fine with having both.

Later she said, "The golden planet in the vision turned blue and green and became the earth. When you worked on my arms it felt like I had my arms wrapped around the earth holding it. This felt so precious and safe and secure."

We talked some more after the session. Anne was still filled with joy and gratitude for ZB, for the people she has met doing ZB and for the richness it has brought to her life. I worked with her for a while to help her fully let in the feeling of gratitude and feel the full impact that ZB has had on her life. Over the last several years I have studied a form of psychotherapy called AEDP (Accelerated Experiential Dynamic Psychotherapy, founded by Diana Fosha). This training has been a major boost to my ability to help clients with deep emotions. I have learned so much from that training, but one major thing I have learned from that training is to help the client feel the full impact of what has just happened.

I also learned to let myself feel the full impact of the client on me. Being more aware of my own experience softens me and lets me feel more compassion for, and more connected to, my clients. Once I am aware of my feelings, I have a choice of how to use that information. I can choose to judiciously let them know how I am impacted when I feel it is appropriate. Done in the right way, this can make a big impression on the client and build deeper trust and deeper connection, which in turn allows more change to happen. In this case I shared with Anne how moved I was by all she had gone through and all she was feeling. I told her how glad and grateful I was to work with her and how happy it made me to see her happiness. Saying this solidified a bond between us. She in turn felt grateful to me, and I think that helped her to do even more deep work the next time we met.

Chapter 7
Creating a Frame

Walter is a male in his fifties working in the health field. He had been coming to see me for Zero Balancing sporadically for a few years, always to work on self-actualization rather than particular physical symptoms. He was interested not only in feeling good and expansive but also in learning more about himself. He had started coming in more regularly as he wanted to make some major progress on issues that were bothering him.

In Zero Balancing we always start talking with the person with a process we call *framing*. This really means asking what are their goals for today's session, but calling it a frame brings to mind a picture frame with four sides creating a container for what is said and done. The benefit of a container is that is can amplify what is inside, just like a pressure cooker can build up heat and energy. Food cooked in a pressure cooker will cook in far shorter time that it would take if it were cooked in a pot with no lid. So one purpose of the frame is to amplify what is said and give it more power, both for the client and the practitioner. In ZB we believe that anything said out loud to another person begins to set things in motion and actually makes it more likely to happen.

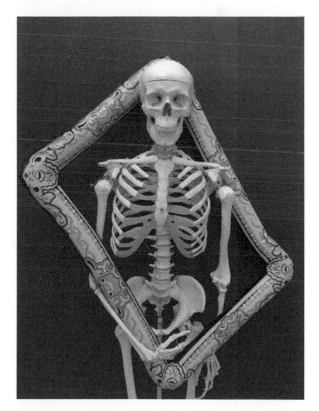

Fig. 7.1

We use Framing in Zero Balancing to clarify and amplify the goals for the ZB session.

(Photo: James McCormick.)

Some clients will have a physical frame. They may have back pain or headaches or foot pain and their whole frame is to get relief from those pains. This is totally fine, and some ZB sessions are about relieving those kinds of symptoms. On the other hand, we can encourage a client also to have a larger frame for a ZB session. This can be a frame that seeks change not only physically but also mentally or emotionally or even spiritually. ZB sessions can help a person access those levels, and as clients get accustomed to the process of Zero Balancing, they come to look forward to the framing as an important part of the process.

Doug, in the first case history in the book, had a frame, which was "Help to remove my doubt." One client came to me years ago asking me to "help restore my faith." Many people have a frame of wanting to get in touch with and live from their "core self." Someone might have a frame to "help me let go of my anger." So frames can be anything that is important to the person, and ZB can often help with those types of requests by freeing up the held energy that is preventing these changes from happening spontaneously.

One notable use of framing, in my own ZB experience, was a series of sessions designed to help me deal with my fear of heights. I was going on a trip to Peru. I had already been there once, and had felt a lot of fear of the heights in a few different situations on the trip. This time I wanted to deal with my fears ahead of time so they weren't so prevalent. In every ZB session I had for six months before the trip, I had, as my main frame, to lessen or remove my fear of heights. The only other thing I did was to go to the top of the tallest buildings in Boston and look down over the side and let myself feel whatever fears I had. But I only did this once. The main thing I did was use the frame in ZB sessions. I didn't know the result until I arrived in Peru, and I found that I was much less afraid.

When a client has a goal of doing personal work and personal exploration, the framing process becomes even more important. One day Walter came in for a ZB session, and we started the framing process with a long talk about how he was feeling frustrated. He was feeling bad about himself for not having the words to describe to me how had he felt after his ZB session the week before. He felt that he was "letting me down." He was directing a lot of negativity toward himself, which was a common experience for him. The good part about it was that the process of framing led him to think more about the right words and about what had actually happened. The words he finally came up with for what he felt were "wrong" and "no." These words epitomized exactly the issue he was dealing with, feeling that somehow he had done the wrong thing and therefore he was "wrong."

He began to talk about his love and hate for his father. He felt that his father loved him but was unable to say it or put it into words and unable to convey these feelings in other ways. I said to Walter, "This all seems very delicate to you," by which I meant that his sense of self-esteem was very tied into these thoughts and feelings. He agreed. He felt bad about himself for having negative feelings about his father. It was usually too painful to let someone see these negative feelings, as well as how bad he felt for having them.

As we talked, I helped him to tolerate the whole range of feelings, to continue to feel them and not run away from them. He told me when I was working on his pelvis in the previous ZB session, he'd had a series of strong images of his father bending over him trying to do an unspecified ritual of some sort, a rite or ritual that was very important to Walter's development. But his father had thick gloves on his hands and something over his head that made it awkward for him to feel or to see. So through no fault of his own, his father couldn't do the job correctly. He didn't have the right equipment. Because of that, the ritual wasn't done correctly and Walter was somehow "compromised." Something that he needed. and should have had, wasn't given to him, and thus his whole life had felt compromised since that time.

These images came to him during the last ZB session, and captured the issue he had been dealing with his whole life. He had been feeling "compromised or not complete or not able to do things right." He had always had strong feelings of letting his father down, mixed with anger at his father not being able to do the ritual correctly. So it became complicated and layered. His father was "wrong" and had "failed" Walter, and at the same time Walter was "wrong" because he never got what he needed to be whole and complete, and also because he had such negative feelings towards his father for compromising him.

We set the frame for this session as, "To help you get outside your early conditioning of being compromised, so you can feel complete and okay about yourself."

This is a great example of a frame in Zero Balancing that goes way beyond the physical aspects of the client and includes his personality, emotional state and energetic state. Having a broad frame like this gives the session a running start. The realizations the client has while talking allows shift in the physical body to happen before we ever get to the table. The ZB session can have a deeper effect on the person and help create change at a more fundamental level, where some of the emotional baggage has been stored in his body.

Some of the hurts we endure in our lives get fully processed by our psyches and don't seem to leave much of a negative imprint. Other hurts are bigger than we can manage, and the feelings that don't get fully processed get stored in the body. As was said in the last chapter, in Zero Balancing we especially look for the effects of the hurts that are stored in the bones. Our clinical experience has shown us that some of our deepest unresolved traumas are housed in our bones. These appear as tension, knots, dullness, resistance and other distortions in the quality of the bones themselves. Freeing the energy in the bones allows the body to process the old hurt in the present, and this can help to free us from some early conditioning. Many people are amazed, and even incredulous, that we can aim for this type of change with Zero Balancing, but the truth is that we see it all the time. We believe that freeing the energy held in the bones allows these old wounds to be more fully processed and integrated in ways that leave both our bodies and our minds more balanced and healthy. The picture below gives a graphic look at how this might happen from a fulcrum into a bone.

In this session, the framing led to a highly successful ZB session. We did a full ZB, and Walter went into a deep state very quickly. He became still and calm early on in the session. He felt in touch with a deep part of himself that he hadn't experienced before this. He had a lot of working signs, indicative of significant personal change and of being in an altered state of consciousness. Walter's working signs were mostly deep breaths, but also rapid eyelid flutters and a tremulous slight shaking of his head. Other than these slight movements, he was extremely still. His field was quiet, almost as if all his atoms and molecules had come to rest.

Over the last few sessions before this one, I had seen how much Walter was holding in his body. There were a lot of places where some movement was possible and would happen, but then I would run into resistance. I was aware of him not wanting to go into certain feelings. This session

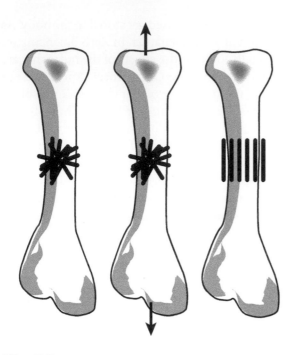

Fig. 7.2

When there is held energy in a bone the tissue can get distorted. The picture on the left lets you imagine how the distorted tissue might look like pick-up-sticks when they are first thrown down. They are very disorganized. The middle picture shows the same bone with traction being applied to both ends of the bone. This traction creates an energy field in the bone and causes the disorganized tissue to realign more towards normal, which you can see in the last picture on the right. The tissue has become aligned (like iron filings over a magnet) and you can get the idea that the bone on the right will more easily move energy through its structure. Any time we put traction, torsion or compression on a bone we create this kind of organizing field which helps to disperse bone held vibration and lead to feelings of energy, lightness and connection.

(Credit: James McCormick.)

was different. There was more movement and thus more softness in all the tissues, and thus more change. The experience of sharing strong feelings during the framing had made it easier for his body to shift. The shift had already begun before I touched him. There was less need for him to hide or protect, which allowed his body to change, and this in turn allowed his emotions to change. As the session went on he said he felt "awesome and present and good." He was clearly not still identified with the belief that he was "bad."

Walter lay on the table a long time after the session, without moving. He was feeling extremely peaceful and extraordinarily good about himself. He felt complete, not compromised. I left him in that place without asking him to describe the sensations he was having. I suggested he "stay with the experience of the feeling in his body," not the words. I wanted him to take in the feeling of being complete. I didn't want him to get caught in the words or in trying to explain it to me. I could always hear about it the next time I saw him.

Once the frame is in place for a session, we specifically ask the client not to *work* on the frame as they receive the session. We don't want them trying to figure out the solution to the issue, because thinking (rather than feeling) can block energetic movement. Similarly, and maybe counter-intuitively, we also suggest the practitioner not dwell on the frame during the session. We want the ZBer also to be in touch with what she feels and not too involved in the thinking side of the brain. As the session goes along, there may be a place where a thought about the frame pops into the head of the ZBer, and she may do something to strengthen or activate the desire expressed in the frame. But the ZBer isn't supposed to spend the whole session thinking about it. We ask both practitioner and client to let the process happen, and with a good connected ZB session a lot of it *will* happen.

In this case, I did not have to do something extra to help Walter's frame happen. He was so ready to change, from the work we had done in other sessions, that during this session he began to change and open right away. As we went along it was clear he was beginning to feel good about himself and beginning to get outside his early conditioning. I just kept doing good connected ZB and allowing his body and energy to open.

Chapter 8
Living From Your Core Self

There are many different therapeutic and spiritual systems that work with the idea that there is a *core self* inside each person, which is always perfect and always with us. Our task is not so much to develop that self as to uncover it. In this process we uncover and lessen the conditioning and beliefs and behaviors that keep us from being aware of that self.

I believe in the idea of the core self and personally want to live from that place in my own life as much as possible. I heard Ben Lipton, an Accelerated Experiential Dynamic Psychotherapy (AEDP) faculty member in New York, express it as "being in that place where everything about us feels right and true." When we are in that place, there is much less need for thinking or worrying. Even the difficult times are easier. When I am there I feel as if "there is nothing to do." This doesn't mean that I am not doing anything, but I don't *need* to do anything, and much more of my awareness is on just being.

It seems that my core self has no age and feels the same now as it did when I was a child. It also feels as if that self has its own consciousness and own directions, and often what I call "me," the ego self, is just along for the ride. Father Claude Larre, now deceased, was a classical Chinese scholar who possessed great knowledge and great joy. He translated an early Chinese saying, "Life is spoken of as a rambling walk where we are guided appropriately if we let the Spirits lead the parade and take us with them."

Richard Schwartz (Schwartz, 1995), the originator of a psychotherapy style called Internal Family Systems, lists some of the qualities we see in people who live from their core selves:

"Curiosity, courage, compassion, creativity, confidence, clarity, connectedness, commitment to service, flow, lightness, openness, acceptance and presence. Others feel at ease with him or her. They have a passion for life, a sense of freedom, a lack of a need for self-promotion. Their eyes, body language and energy all say they are authentic, solid and unpretentious." It's an impressive list.

The following case history shows a client feeling out of touch with her core self, and not even sure she has one. Ronnie is a long term client in her seventies. At one point in her life she was a nun and later on a massage therapist. She had taken a few ZB classes, so she was familiar with the process and the possibilities of Zero Balancing.

41

Ronnie came in feeling a bit lost for this session. She felt out of touch with herself and sensed that something was "missing." She has often felt that in her life. She was adopted, and her adoptive father died when she was very young. She was moved around a great deal as a child, living with different parts of her family and in a foster home. She always felt she didn't have the right role model. She always felt she had missed getting "some important information that everyone else had." This led to her feeling that she didn't know "what to do in my life or how to move ahead." She thought she didn't have what she needed and that she should "create a self."

I told her she didn't need to create a self. I suggested that she did have a clear, full, excellent core self already and that all she had to do was to tune in to that self. Together we decided the frame for the session would be to help her connect to her core self.

After some further discussion, and before we went to the table to begin the ZB session, I asked Ronnie to tune in to her body and see what she noticed. She went to a place of anxiety in her upper abdomen just under the xiphoid process, below her sternum. She felt a "burning hot hole" there. To me this was hugely significant. Ronnie was describing a very strong field of energy in her chest. Experience has shown that exploring this type of sensation usually produces profound insight and change for the client.

I wanted to bring more of her attention, and more of my attention, to that place. We could have done a lot of work right there while we were still sitting and talking, but I decided to go ahead and begin the session and work with that area while she was on the table. To start the session, I put my hands on her shins as I often do, and just listened without trying to do anything other than feel the state of her energetic field in the bones. What

I felt was an energy that I described as "anxiety that was looking around slightly in panic, not sure what to do with itself." I know Ronnie well and felt comfortable enough with her to describe what I was feeling.

She replied with what she felt in her abdomen, an "anxiety whirling around." So we were on the same wavelength and I felt strongly connected to her and her donkey. I asked her to tune in to that feeling of anxiety and to feel it and pay attention to it without trying to change it. She was able to do that, and once she did, she immediately began to feel it change.

After touching her shins and doing the initial half moon of the session, I asked Ronnie if I could touch the area of the "burning hole" she had mentioned before. I put one finger on the area under her xiphoid process. I was holding light pressure there, and just with that light contact she and I both felt things shift. Then she felt the burning get less, and I could feel that whirling, panicky energy lessen.

As things were shifting, Ronnie started talking about how her grandmother had said to her that she was "cracked" in her upper back. I wasn't sure what that meant but I decided to look for that place in her back. I found the place with my left hand where she felt cracked, on the spine in between the third and fourth thoracic vertebrae. I put one hand gently there, in touch with the bones of the spine, and kept one finger on the "burning hole" in the front. She immediately felt that these two places connected to each other, and she felt really good when I touched both of them at the same time.

I held them both for several minutes (which I've mentioned before is a long time for Zero Balancing). As I kept holding the touch, the sensation of the burning hole kept spreading out and smoothing out. She had the sense of the "holes" in her "filling up," which was a relief and felt wonderful to her. The feeling of filling up physically was also filling up her sense of herself.

Her sensations kept shifting to the point that the feeling of the burning hole was almost entirely gone. As that happened she began to smile, to feel more relaxed and to feel more connected to herself. By the end of the session she was no longer having the feeling of emptiness or of something missing. Instead she became aware of the fullness of her experience and of herself. I asked how that felt and she said it felt "freeing" and "great" and that she did feel "connected to herself." She felt in touch with her essence, and that allowed her to feel at home, to feel right. The questions of what to do were no longer even relevant.

We talked about how that experience is always available to her and reminded her that she does have a strong core self. She just has to remember to tune in to it and check in to herself. Ronnie said she felt grateful and now saw the feeling of "missing something" as an old habit not based on current reality. When she felt in touch with her own sensations, she felt whole. This made her hopeful and happy. The hope was that she could live in a way that kept her connected to herself, helped her feel whole and helped her feel well.

This is a great example of one of my basic aims with Zero Balancing, which is to help people live from the core self more of the time, where it is much smoother surfing. In addition to whatever symptoms a person might want to have addressed with a ZB session, I always hope to encourage this connection. And one way to get there is to help the client learn to pay attention to her bodily experience. Each time a person discovers the core self, it gets easier and easier to make that discovery again.

Another example of getting in touch with the core self occurred in a session with Maria. Maria is an artist with a history of receiving and doing personal work through yoga, meditation and Zero Balancing sessions. In her last few sessions we had aimed at helping her stay connected with her core self. In this session we settled on a frame of continuing to help her feel more in contact with her core self.

During the framing, we talked about issues that came from her past, with her mother – Maria's feelings of being overly rigid and aggressive, of standing tall to ward off inner feelings of collapse, of not being enough. Frequently in her life, she felt bad about herself, and her guilt and grief had led to her wanting to give up.

At one point as we talked, she let herself physically collapse, and she realized there were some benefits to doing that. She felt relief and relaxation, less burdened, less pressured to hold herself up. It was actually much easier. Allowing herself to collapse with awareness had a number of good qualities.

I started the session and immediately, with the first touch on her shins, I could feel her core energetic self. It felt strong and clear and easy to access. When I did the half moon vector at her feet, I felt the same energy. I held the half moon a long time to amplify and anchor her experience of being in touch with her core self.

As I moved to the pelvis, again I had the sense of being in touch with a deep part of her, a part I thought she was also in touch with, though I couldn't be sure. I told her what I was doing. I wouldn't do this with everyone, but she had a lot of ZB and meditation experience and could use the information. I thought it would benefit her and allow her to connect more fully to that part of herself.

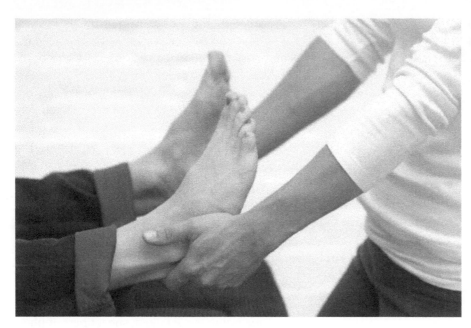

Fig. 8.1

Half moon vector at the feet.

(Photo: Tom Gentile.)

I said, "My job is to help you get in touch with the energetic signature of your core self, to make it stronger, and to hold you in that energetic experience for a long time. This will help anchor it in your body and in your consciousness."

She said, "How do you know it's my core self? What does it feel like to you?"

I said the energy felt "clear, strong, pure, alive and has sparkle or effervescence." Those words did help her tune in to that part.

As the session went on I continued to feel the same sensations most of the time. I felt them also in her hip fulcrums and in the feet fulcrums. I also noticed a tendency (mild in this session, though it had been much stronger at times in the past) to pull away from the core, as if it was too scary or overwhelming. At a couple of points in the session, Maria did have emotions rise to the surface. One time it was grief, another time, anxiety. Both of these were strong enough to be unsettling to her but didn't last long, and Maria

was able to re-connect with her core feelings as the session went on.

When I worked with her upper body, initially it was not as easy to access her core field. She was more defended in her upper back and neck, and things moved more slowly. But if I also moved slowly and held fulcrums longer, we could both feel that clear feeling. She said she felt energetic movement in her lower body increasing as we worked with the upper body, and she felt a lot happening in her abdomen. She kept putting her hands there and wondering what exactly she was feeling there. She said it felt kind of hollow and somewhat strange, but also kind of good. I wasn't exactly sure what to make of that sensation, but kept an eye on it. She continued to have that sensation for five to ten minutes.

When I finally got to her head, there was one major blocked space in her neck, between the first cervical vertebra and the skull. There should be a fluid gliding motion between these two bones, and it was almost completely restricted. There is a special fulcrum called the *nod yes fulcrum*, which works to free up this articulation. It involves the client moving the chin up and down, with resistance from the ZBer. After I did that fulcrum with Maria, that joint was completely open. This is often a major opening when the area has been held tightly, and this fulcrum added a major shift to what had already been a big session. The fulcrum allowed her field to expand further and allowed her to feel lighter, more open, more clear and more connected to her feelings.

As I did the closing fulcrums of the session, I felt her field, which had already been strong and clear, get even more full, with more breadth and depth. Her energetic field was more three dimensional, more vibrant.

After the session, when I asked her how she was feeling, she said almost exactly those same words. She felt her energetic field get bigger and broader and fuller. This felt wonderful to her, and she came off the table feeling able to take up her appropriate space. She felt taller and more powerful. And this power was not a forced power but a relaxed presence.

She said, "That was amazing. Can all ZBers do that?" I said the ones with a lot of experience can. She had achieved her goal of feeing more in touch with her core self. And we both felt better. I felt good about my part in what we had achieved, and I also felt clearer and more centered in my core. Whenever the client has a big opening, my system responds to that and I feel better.

Chapter 9
Body Felt Sense

I believe the term *body felt sense* was first used by psychotherapist Dr Eugene Gendlin in his book *Focusing*, published in 1978. I have found the technique of focusing invaluable for helping people make changes in their behavior and their symptoms. It works beautifully with Zero Balancing.

Dr Gendlin writes that a *body felt sense* is a "kind of bodily awareness that profoundly influences our lives. It is not a mental experience but a physical experience. A bodily awareness of a situation or person or an event." (Gendlin, 1978)

Among other things, Dr Gendlin discovered that those psychotherapy patients who had access to this part of themselves were more successful in psychotherapy. They were the ones who changed the most in positive ways. He found that people who did not have access to that part of themselves did not accomplish as much.

This internal bodily awareness is vital in Zero Balancing. ZB is a process that has a lot of potential for helping the person develop conscious access to her own felt sense.

The person I am going to tell you about was a young woman, in her thirties, in graduate school. Paying attention to what was happening in her body quickly improved her symptoms and her

mood, and she began to get useful information from her body.

Olivia came in feeling terrible. She had a long list of things that were bothering her, physical and emotional. She had a number of pain symptoms, including headaches, which she had at the moment she arrived. She had very painful cramps with her period, with bad PMS including depression, back pain and joint pain.

She had Restless Leg Syndrome in her left leg, "so bad I am afraid to go to bed... It's hard for me to breathe. I have an empty feeling in my chest." She was angry, despondent and depressed. She was also severely constipated.

As we talked she added, "I'm a bad person." She meant it and felt it strongly, though to me she clearly was not. "I have the stress of my job getting to me. I am getting ready to present at an important meeting. I hate it. I think I'm bad at my job. Plus, I have to deal with all the stress of holidays. I'm miserable."

All of this poured out of her when I asked the question, "How can I help you?" There was so much worry and so much emotion that it felt like we needed to help her calm down to accomplish anything.

A great way to help people calm down and center is to ask them, "What do you feel in your body?" This causes people to check into their bodies and look for that felt sense. What are the sensations in their bodies? Some people can do this quite easily and give great detail about what they feel. Others very quickly return to their thinking and start to give answers from their thinking rather than from what they feel physically. These people can learn to feel in their bodies, but it takes time to teach them. They need to learn where to look, the value of looking and how to develop the courage to stay with what they feel, even when it doesn't feel good.

In this session, before we did any treatment I asked Olivia to check into her body and see what she felt. She was actually quite good at it and could tune in easily. According to her, she had an empty feeling in her chest and a brick in her lower abdomen. I asked her to stay with the feeling of emptiness in her chest.

In order to get useful information from the body, we have to approach it in a certain way. Dr Gendlin suggests how to do this (Gendlin, 1978). First of all, we ask the client not to try to change anything. She is not to try to make it better, just to feel what is there.

Secondly, she should be as non-judgmental as possible. Ask her to be as curious and as friendly as possible towards what she feels, so she can simply be with it and be connected. The goal is to help her connect to the feeling rather than condemn it, or herself.

Lastly, she needs to have the courage to tolerate whatever feeling is there and to stay with it for a period of time. Sometimes what people feel is good and happy and that is easier to stay with, though sometimes even that will cause difficulties. But if the person feels pain, emptiness, bitterness, rage and disappointment, it is harder to accept and allow and stay with those feelings.

Olivia was able to tolerate her rather strong feelings pretty well. After I asked her to stay with the emptiness, she closed her eyes and listened internally and immediately felt sad. I asked what she was sad about, and she said she felt "lonely and that I am missing something." She began to cry but continued to pay attention to her inner world for a while as she cried. She said she began to feel "warmth" in the formerly empty place.

She continued to pay attention even longer, and she began to feel this warmth coming from her lower abdomen up to the empty place in her chest. Her chest began to feel warm and full and good. Her lower abdomen began to have movement and to feel better as well. So merely the act of paying attention to her *body felt sense*, without judgment and without trying to change what she felt, helped her to feel much better in both mind and body, before we even did any ZB.

I began the session of ZB on Olivia's upper back and neck, which is unusual. I hardly ever start on the upper body in ZB. Because Olivia had such a strong sense in her upper body of emptiness and sadness, I wanted to start the session on her posterior ribs.

I found a place of tension in one rib and asked her to tune in to that rib using the focusing techniques. As I held the pressure of my fulcrum, she kept her attention on what she felt in that spot. We did this on several ribs, and as we did, the tension she had in her ribs got better and better.

The session was going well, but nonetheless, I knew there was more I could do for her. I knew I could help free her of some more of that tension in her ribs and help her get to more freedom and positive feeling for herself.

So I used another part of the focusing techniques and suggested to Olivia that she ask the

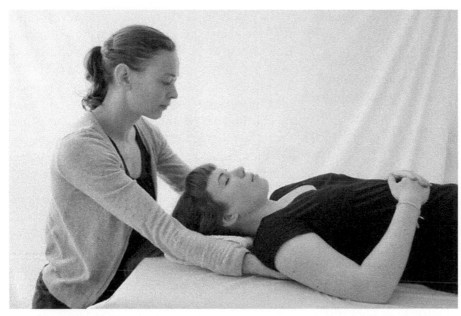

Fig. 9.1

Working with the posterior rib cage in Zero Balancing.

(Photo: Kathryn McNeils.)

rib we were currently working on if it had any information for her. She took a little time with her eyes closed, paying attention, and then opened her eyes and said her rib told her that she needed to keep paying attention to that rib. "It had been feeling bad and was needing attention." (It's important in this kind of exercise, when the person is asking the body rib for information, that the answer come from the body and not the mind. We want the client to get in touch with the wisdom of the body, which is often different from what the client is thinking.)

I went to another rib, which was also holding tension. As I put in the fulcrum and held it, things began to change in this rib as well. As the practitioner, I can feel a myriad of different possible sensation in the rib – softening is a common feeling, where the rib literally changes its consistency. I might feel a rib getting livelier, waking up, or a rib getting fuller or more energetic.

As I felt the change happening, I asked her to do a similar process as the one she had done with the last rib. I wanted her to ask if there was

information. This rib said to "relax and chill." She was doing a good job. "Do not worry about that."

We kept working, and as we worked, Olivia's headache cleared, her breathing deepened and her mood improved. By the end of the session she was smiling, feeling good and feeling no pain.

Olivia felt very well by the end, both physically and mentally. She was grateful. And she had learned an important principle of healing: going into the feeling, not away from it, will often shift the feeling – especially when you go into it without trying to change it, with compassion and curiosity. Looking for her body felt sense, and the information from that place in her body, was very valuable. She had learned how to tune into this for more information whenever she wanted.

I use this technique of asking people to tune into their bodies with a high percentage of people. It is so valuable in helping to guide them to deeper change and deeper connection to their core selves. It's also helpful to me in seeing where they need the most help. There are hundreds of cases I could cite where this has been hugely valuable.

One other that comes to mind is a woman also in her thirties, a human-relations professional. Lillian came in feeling very bad. Or maybe more accurately, not feeling anything at all. The impression I got when I saw her was that she looked like a wilted plant, with all the leaves drooping. When I asked her to check into herself, she was not really in touch with herself or her feelings. She didn't even feel empty. She just felt nothing.

It is counterintuitive to many people, but even when you don't feel anything, if you stay with that experience it will evolve into something else. In this case I asked Lillian to pay attention to her chest and torso even though she initially felt nothing and to notice what happened if she did this with compassion and without trying to change anything.

It took a few minutes but gradually she began to feel sensations in her chest. At first she felt tightness and constriction. As she noticed this sensation, she noticed her breath was also changing by getting more labored. Soon she began to feel more sensation and emotion – sadness – which she felt as a tight band in her chest. I asked her to continue to feel that sensation, without trying to change it and without trying to get rid of it. I asked to see if she could just feel it, accept it and even appreciate it.

She gradually began to feel more sadness, during which time the constriction got even tighter. Then after a while she burst into tears and at that point the constriction began to loosen. Finally, she was able to feel all she had been holding back, unbeknownst to herself. She began to talk a lot about losing her relationship and the pain of that. She felt quite free to talk at this point, and as she did, she cried a lot, and after that she began to feel much better.

I saw Lillian many times over a few years and we almost always went through a similar pattern, where at first she would either say she felt fine or felt nothing, but after I gave her time to tune in to her body, she would invariably get sad. Frequently this revolved around being lonely and wanting a relationship. She would often say, "Why haven't I had a relationship? What's wrong with me?"

If we stayed with her body felt sense, as her awareness of her body increased, her feelings began to change each time. Her thoughts also changed, and she would come out of each session feeling relaxed and expanded. She would be having positive thoughts about herself and the possibilities in her life. Over many sessions, Lillian became more able to incorporate this practice into her life, and her need for external support lessened. She needed less help to stay in touch with her core self and her best self. I have not seen her for over a year now.

Chapter 10
Altered States of Consciousness

One of the hallmarks of Zero Balancing is that we intentionally work with and induce *altered states of consciousness* in the client. As Dr Smith says, through touch we can often help a person drop into a deeper meditative state than she could reach on her own, even after months of meditating. Technically, an altered state of consciousness is any state of awareness that is different from normal waking consciousness. It is a state in which the brain waves have changed.

The *Core Zero Balancing Study Guide* is the teaching manual we use when teaching beginning Zero Balancing classes. The following quote on altered states of consciousness is from the guide:

Expanded states of consciousness

"Brain physiology tells us there are a number of brain wave patterns, each having its own characteristics. In ZB we use 'expanded states of consciousness' or 'altered states of consciousness' to indicate brain waves that move away from a beta, linear-thinking mind set.

Experience has taught us that as people move into expanded states they are less bound by specific definitions of themselves, definitions in which illnesses are often embedded. People seem more prone to change and healing…

Expanded states can be brought about by introducing two contrary sensations simultaneously, such as pain and pleasure, or structure and energy. Holding a fulcrum with these characteristics can induce an expanded state of consciousness, or give the person an experience of unity, which is also an expanded or enhanced awareness."
(Sullivan & Smith, 2020)

As mentioned earlier, we live simultaneously in the world of duality, our normal waking consciousness of everyday reality, and the world of unity, where we feel connected both to our core and to the universe. In this second state, time can seem to stop. In Zero Balancing we can help the client enter into that world of unity consciousness. We can do that through touch in a ZB session by holding our fulcrum for a longer time while keeping awareness of both structure and their energy.

This has a number of different effects in a ZB session. The client's awareness goes more to his internal sensations and not into contact with the outside world. Often the client will report little or no sense of time or space. The client is less tightly bound to his or her normal belief systems or to his sense of who they are, and thus more change is possible. They are able to get outside their normal conditioning.

In the introduction I mentioned the research completed in March 2017, carried out by the Zero Balancing Touch Foundation, that studied the effects of ZB sessions on clients. At the end of that study we also did a pilot study with subjects wearing EEG monitors while receiving Zero Balancing sessions. The preliminary findings showed a great deal of change in the brain waves of clients, potentially indicating they had gone into altered states of consciousness. This matches our clinical experience and was enough evidence for us to plan a larger study of the effects of ZB on the brain waves of clients.

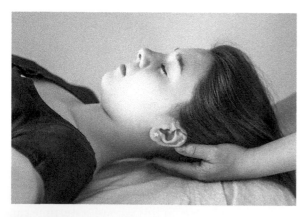

Fig. 10.1

The serenity of a client in an altered state.

(Image: iStock-180829725.jpg)

A good example of a client going into an altered state through Zero Balancing is a session with Brian, a Zero Balancing faculty member in his fifties. We had done many ZB sessions together. On this day, a third of the way into a ZB session I began to do a fulcrum we call the lateral leg fulcrum, coming down the side of the leg from the hip joint along the *tensor fasciae latae* muscle. I took a long time doing this fulcrum, much longer than usual. I kept the connection very clear and kept moving more and more slowly as I went down his leg.

When you do this fulcrum slowly, and then more and more slowly as you go, the client will often start to experience time shifting. The person receiving the ZB can go into an altered state of consciousness where time stands still or is irrelevant. The person is so involved in his internal experience, there is almost no sense of the outside world. A client in that state of awareness is more able to change his beliefs, his physical body and his attitudes. Brian is a very experienced ZB practitioner and a very experienced meditator. He was able to go with this strong slow influence and allow his awareness to shift.

There are signs that indicate a person is in an altered state. The breathing usually changes, developing either a prolonged shallow breath or a number of deep breaths. The pulse often gets stronger, and you can see the pulse in the aorta in the throat beating strongly. You can sometimes see the heart beat in the whole rib cage. With Brian, all these things were happening as I came down his leg from the hip to the ankle.

As the fulcrum continued, I moved more and more slowly and his breathing deepened more. He began having deeper breaths and more frequent breaths. I could feel in my hands the intensity of his energy building and getting stronger.

I began to feel in my body what was happening for him. My own energy field began to get stronger and to pulsate more. It was building so much that I was having trouble tolerating the surge of energy. I realized that I had to expand my field and go past my own limitations to allow him to shift as fully as he was able.

I needed to relax more and to breathe and let my own system adjust to the new input. I had to be careful not to let my limitations shut him down, which would happen if I couldn't allow the expansion in myself. Soon, I was able to let my energy expand, and he was able to keep going. The internal change in him kept growing.

It brought tears to his eyes, tears of joy, and also tears of mourning for not having this experience all the time. This continued for the rest of the session.

When we finished the session, Brian's eyes were bright. He felt alert, energized and yet relaxed. He felt grateful for our connection and for the work in general. He said he was "able to experience the world in a new way." He had received many ZB sessions from skilled practitioners, but he felt this was the best and deepest experience he'd had of that fulcrum. The experience left us both feeling connected to each other, expanded and filled with love for each other.

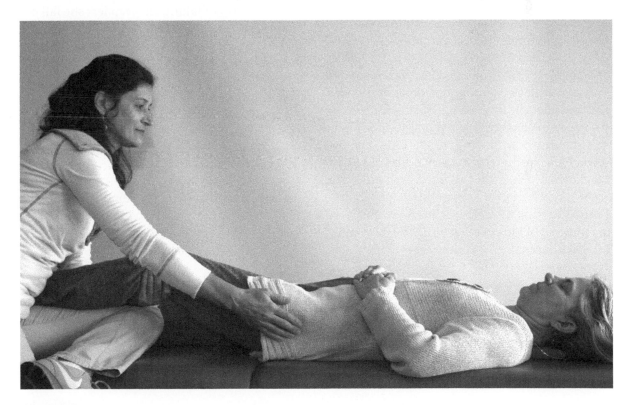

Fig. 10.2

Fulcrum from the hip joint and down the side of the gall bladder meridian.

(Photo: Giovanni Pescetto.)

This ability of Zero Balancing sessions to help a person move into expanded states of consciousness is one of the main reasons we talk about Zero Balancing as a body and mind system that facilitates personal transformation. Clients that have this type of experience begin to experience the world in new ways. Their early conditioning is lessened, and their perceptions become clearer and less clouded by their past history.

Another example of an altered state from Zero Balancing was described in the preface with Ella, who was in a deep altered state in that session. As I wrote, "Ella's bones and the soft tissues literally felt livelier, more elastic, and more vibrant, and similarly her energetic field became more lively and sparkly. And in between these movements she would have periods of extreme stillness, her body not moving while her energetic field grew quieter and quieter. We talked for thirty minutes after the session. She was very animated during this time. She looked, and said she felt, totally alive. As she felt this joy, she began to connect to her younger self who, she remembered, was 'smiling all the time.' She had a beautiful expression of amazement on her face at the experience she'd just had. She felt 'refreshed and renewed… I feel alive like I haven't felt for decades… I can't stop smiling. I feel so much joy it's almost bursting out of me... I feel new… I feel surprised… I feel like dancing… I have a swagger to me.'"

In another session with Ella, she again went into a deep altered state. She told me afterwards about her experience during the session. "During the early part of the session I saw a large, round, glass bowl with very dirty water in it. The water gradually became clearer and clearer, and then was totally clear. Then there was a goldfish swimming in the bowl. And finally I was the goldfish, happily and easily swimming in the clear water in the sunshine."

Finally, another client, Rita, had an experience that she told me about after the session. During the early part of the session she felt she was walking on a tightrope with a blindfold and no net, fearful of taking any step lest she fall off. As the session progressed, she realized that she could take the blindfold off. So she saw herself and felt herself still on the tightrope, but at least she could now see, which was much safer. Near the end of the session she had a vision of herself, no longer with the blindfold, and able to step off the tightrope. She was on the ground in no danger, with a clear vision of herself and her life.

These are all examples of the kinds of experiences people have when they are able to allow their consciousness to drop in to an altered state. Zero Balancing can help that process happen.

Chapter 11
Verbal Fulcrums

It is not always necessary to do a lot of talking with a ZB session. It often goes beautifully and works on a deep part of the person without any verbal processing. Nonetheless, as we have seen in this book, there are situations where verbally working with the client can add whole new dimensions to the process and allow outcomes that would not have happened with the bodywork alone.

I have created a Zero Balancing course entitled *Verbal Fulcrums in Zero Balancing*, which emphasizes the importance of counseling, or processing, and begins to teach Zero Balancers how to develop the necessary skills. My intention in this chapter is to give an example of how the verbal part of any therapeutic interaction can be extremely important to the outcome. As UK psychiatrist Michael Balint said, "If doctors in their practices did not respond to and work with the psychological implications of what was happening for their patients, it was a major missed opportunity." I think the same is true of Zero Balancing sessions, and the session below is a good example of how processing can add a great deal of value to a ZB session.

Cassandra is a young consultant, married with two small children. She came in saying she felt both "tired and wired," though her main complaints were physical. She'd had pain in her left lower back around her sacroiliac joint for the last four days. The pain came on suddenly and was at first a 7 out of 10, though it was down to a 4 out of 10. This pain was a mirror image of a pain she felt on her right side from a fall a few months earlier. She also had discomfort in her right shoulder. So the initial frame in this session was to help her with these various pains.

Once I started doing the ZB, it was clear to me her body held a lot of stress and tension. The tissues felt very tight and were not yielding much. As I held the fulcrums, I wasn't feeling much change. I was feeling a lack of movement in the sacroiliac area.

I felt the same lack of movement when I moved on to her hips and feet. But the holding was especially prominent in the area we call the dorsal hinge (the tenth to twelfth ribs in the back). This proved to be major area of release in this session.

It is always a choice in a Zero Balancing session whether or not to mention what I am feeling to the client. If done poorly, the client can feel shamed, and it is easy to lose rapport. In this session with Cassandra, I felt we had a strong

55

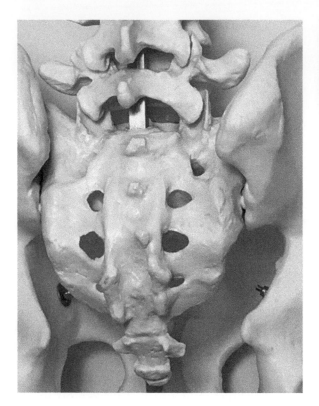

Fig. 11.1

Sacrum and sacroiliac joint. The sacroiliac joint is the main foundation joint in the lower back.

(Photo: James McCormick.)

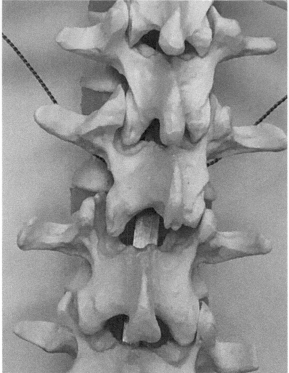

Fig. 11.2

Lumbar vertebrae. In the lumbar area of the spine the articulations where the vertebrae meet each other are nearly vertical. Because of the angle of these articulations, the lumbar vertebrae can flex a lot and extend some but there is very little rotation in these joints.

(Photo: James McCormick.)

enough relationship that I could talk to her about what I was sensing. I said to her, "It seems like your body is holding a lot of tension. It is very tight and not changing very much." Far from being upset, she agreed with this assessment and said she felt very tense. I said, "It seems like there must be a lot of stress in your life at this time." Again she agreed.

As we have talked about earlier in the book, it is possible to feel the quality of what is being held in the tension. With Cassandra, I felt how strongly she was keeping herself tight, and I began

to perceive this was to help her control her feelings and not get overwhelmed. Again I chose to mention this to her. "My perception is that you are holding yourself very tight to keep steady in the face of the stress around you and to give you more sense of control."

Cassandra once again immediately agreed with this statement, but it was new information to her. She hadn't known how much she was holding

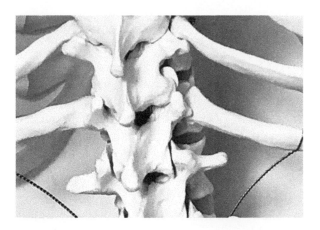

Fig. 11.3

Dorsal hinge. The thoracic vertebrae articulations are oblique and more nearly horizontal. Because of this different angle, these vertebrae allow a lot of rotation, which the lumbar vertebrae do not. Most of this change from vertical to oblique and horizontal happens in one vertebra. The bottom vertebra in this picture is the 12th thoracic rib and shows the bottom facets are vertical (like a lumbar) and the top facets on the same vertebra are oblique (like a thoracic vertebra.) We call this vertebra the dorsal hinge. The effect of this anatomical variation is important for the functioning of the whole lower back.

(Photo: James McCormick.)

or that she was protecting herself so much. This led to a whole new level of dialogue between us, in which she said, "I thought I just came in for a little pain in my back."

As I was working on the ribs in the dorsal hinge area, I asked her to bring her attention to the place where my fingers were in touch with the tension, and to see what she felt there without judgment and without trying to change anything. I asked her to be curious and friendly towards what she

felt. As Cassandra did this, she tuned into a strong tightness in her chest. She talked about feeling a cage around her heart that served to protect her by not letting things move. I asked her to keep her awareness there, and, as she did, for the first time she felt things begin to change. Her breath deepened and the tension began to lessen. The movement was slow, but she said, "It feels better."

At that point I could feel even more clearly what was being held. I said, "I can sense that the opening and lessening of tension feels good, but that there is fear about it. Fear about what else you might feel." She said, "Absolutely, yes, but I didn't know I was such an open book."

I asked what the fear was about, and she said, "Fear of getting into the chaos and a mess and not being able to get out of it." As we worked with this fear, her sadness started to come up. Not deep sadness or tears but sadness that got stronger as we went along.

As the session progressed, Cassandra was gradually becoming more and more open to looking at her deep feelings. This was in part due to the Zero Balancing easing the stress and tension in her body, and also because our verbal connection was letting her feel met and understood. Trust was gradually being built, but was still an issue – trust of me but also of herself. As she had said, she feared getting into some deep emotional place and not being able to get out. I told her, "You have enough skills that you can trust your body to let go and you can deal with whatever comes up. You can feel your sadness and pain and won't have to stay in the sadness and chaos forever."

I began to sense that some of the issues might have to do with her family. I asked, "Is your family involved?" She said yes and was reluctant to talk about it much, but it was clear that some of her sadness had to do with that. She said, "We are trying to work things out."

Cassandra was feeling moved by the quality of the listening she was receiving. She felt cared for, and was grateful to be met and heard. Though she didn't say so, I had a sense she wanted more of that in her life, perhaps from her husband. I left it up to her at this time to decide if she wanted to bring up more issues about her relationship, and she was very circumspect about it.

As we finished the ZB she felt far more relaxed, more able to let down, more able to let things soften in her body. The hard cage she had felt in her chest was much softer. She was still very much in touch with all the feelings that had emerged. She felt more sadness, but she also felt very grateful she had been able to explore those feelings. She had not known all that was going on inside, and the session brought her increased conscious awareness.

She had put a limit on how far she wanted to go that day, but she went pretty far. I appreciated her for being so courageous to let all these feelings emerge. I also gave her some homework – to listen to her body and to trust it as much as she could. I encouraged her to meditate on her body sensations and have a dialogue with herself through her body. I suggested she come back in whenever she chose.

This session demonstrates once again just how much the practitioner can read of the feelings in the client by getting in touch with the tissues and paying attention. It also shows a session where the verbal processing was as important as the bodywork. Cassandra was coming in for her various pains, and by the end of the session, due to the processing we did, she had ventured into a whole new territory that had the potential to benefit her life. And her physical discomfort was much less.

Another really good example of the value of verbal fulcrums in coordination with a ZB session came with Tori. She had received many ZB sessions over a number of years, but this session was particularly noteworthy.

We had a long talk at the beginning of the session – maybe 30 minutes. She talked about how she felt "tired and weighed down" and how the "weight of trying to hold herself up and to live a good life was relentless and hard to bear". At times she "just wanted to give up."

At one point in the conversation I asked her to pay attention to what she was feeling in her body. As she took a minute to pay attention (we had done this many times in the past and she was very open to it and used to it) she said "I feel like collapsing." As she said that she let her body sag. She put her head down and let her shoulders come forward and her chest cave, and was slumping over, physically and also mentally. She was in what looked to me like a defeated posture, and initially felt to her like a defeated posture.

As she stayed in that position she began to talk more. She grew up having to be very strong and rigid to hold her own and be able to resist her mother's will. She had to hold herself up and had become very tired. This pattern was still with her and had been all of her adult life.

Tori continued to allow herself to slump and to continue to pay attention to what she felt in her body while in that position. Gradually, with time, she began to feel some relief and release in her body. She got more relaxed and relieved. She stayed there a long time, and she kept feeling better and better. She felt a big relief of not having to hold herself up and not having to look like she was okay when she didn't feel that way. She began to feel more relaxed, lighter, and then happier. She didn't *have* to hold herself up. She wasn't having to resist being taken over by her mother.

After staying in that position for a long time she began to almost involuntarily straighten up without any effort or force. She began to uncurl and hold her head up with natural ease. She was not rigid, not having to protect herself and just *being* without effort. She had allowed herself to listen to and respond to her inner world and her feeling while doing that was one of joy and accomplishment.

The result of this process was that before we ever got to the table there was already a big shift with both her physical body and her mood. She was feeling much lighter, more relaxed, less effortful and she was happier with more joy and more pride.

This made a huge difference when we went into the ZB session. Doing some verbal processing and framing first allowed the ZB to start from a much more open place and allowed the session to produce a much bigger change than usual.

We made the frame for her Zero Balancing session to help her "to just be, without effort." Tori had already been doing that by the end of the framing so it was more about amplifying that feeling rather than having to create it from scratch. Her energy was much more accessible. Right from my first touch on her shins I felt able to connect to all of her, not just to her shins. The feeling in her field was alive and shimmering, more so than she had been in any previous session. The verbal work had both shifted her body and her energy field, but also connected her much more to herself as well as to me. We both agreed later that this allowed a more powerful session than ever before. We'd had a running start on the session.

The whole ZB went extremely well. She was at ease from the beginning and allowing her body to shift. It wasn't hard for me to follow her lead. She had major working signs throughout the session. The part I remember the most was working with her arms about halfway through the work

on the upper body. In many sessions the arm fulcrums feel good and useful but frequently not the most impactful part of the session. This time was different.

I felt along the upper arm, applying simple fulcrums with pressure and rotation. As I was energetically connecting with both the muscles of the upper arm, the bone gold held in the bone of the humerus and the energy of the whole upper arm, I felt I was talking directly to Tori, not just working with tight tissues. I felt like I was working with her *being* through her arms. It's a little hard to describe but there are times when as the practitioner you feel like you are working locally with muscle and bone, and other times where doing essentially the same motions, you feel you are affecting much more than that local area. The place you are touching the person is much more energetically charged. It feels as if you are tapped into the source, like the faucet was suddenly fully opened and the water poured through.

The field locally got stronger, but it also expanded and felt like it was now affecting the whole body. I could feel it affecting Tori in a deeper way, so not just geographically wider, but more down to the core of the person. And the part of her responding to the touch was different. It was more personal and more emotional with more significant change. In this session the work with Tori's arms was a doorway to more overall change for her both personally and physically.

Often the practitioner can sense this by the client having more working signs. Yet another signal of this change was that I could also feel more happening in my own field. I was being affected by the increased energy. I began to feel more lively, more energized, even happier. Reading the reaction in my own body was a clear message about how the session was proceeding.

After the session she said similar things about the session and about her arms. She felt the whole of her being treated with each part and not just a series of separate parts being treated. And her arms felt particularly that way to her. She, too, felt the work on her arms had been particularly powerful.

All of this led to a very good outcome. Her eyes were very bright at the end. She could actually see more clearly. She held herself up very straight but without any effort. She felt happier and lighter. She didn't have to resist anything and was able to allow herself and her spirits to "lead the parade." The work of allowing herself to collapse in the beginning had led to major change in her ability to "just be" with whatever was happening.

Part Two

Healing Principles

2

Chapter 12
Amplify the Wellness

We have talked a lot in the earlier cases about ZB sessions aimed at helping someone ease suffering or pain or the impact of difficult emotions. This is not, however, the only way of helping people with Zero Balancing. Just as powerful as easing or removing blocked energy, which causes pain, is the ability to amplify what feels good in the person. Sometimes we talk of amplifying the wellness.

It is one our basic beliefs in Zero Balancing, supported by our clinical experience, that we can find the vibration of every part of the person somewhere in his energetic field. The metaphor that comes to mind is when physicists can still find the vibration of the big bang, now thought to be 13 billion years ago, in the universe. The imprint is still there in all that exists today. In a similar way, all of our earlier experiences leave a bodily and energetic imprint somewhere in our systems.

Just as we can find the evidence of an earlier trauma in the bones and in the energy of the person, we can also always find the "wellness" in the person's vibration, even if he has numerous ailments now. Sometimes we can choose to work "beneath the illness." If we can find that healthy vibration, we can boost it. With someone who carries trauma, we can try to find the part that existed before the trauma. Or in a person with a current illness, we can find within him the healthy part. This can help the person by giving him more energy, more hope and more perspective on his current situation, which allows more movement to happen within the ill part as well.

In a style of psychotherapy I have been studying for the last two years, Accelerated Experiential Dynamic Psychotherapy (AEDP), one of the basic tenets is to "privilege the positive." There are numerous reasons for this, one of which is that it starts to free up the person. Helping him get in touch with his positive feelings and experiences often gives him more resources with which to work on the more challenging feelings. We can do this same thing directly with the body.

Walter is a regular, though infrequent, client of Zero Balancing. (We met him earlier in Chapter 7 on Framing.) He came in for his session on this day with a slightly wild look on his face. I usually see him as a calm, spiritual man with some anxiety, but not overly scattered. But that day was different.

His eyes were shining in an almost manic state (though he is not manic-depressive.) He talked rapidly about his worries including his high cholesterol counts and other blood tests. He talked about how two to three drinks a night helped him calm down. He had not spoken of this before, so it was new information to me. I wasn't sure if this was just recent or had been going on for a long time.

He was on day nineteen of a meditation practice to help calm him, which he felt good about but seemed to me to be only mildly helpful. He was still very revved up. He talked of strain at work and the tensions and nervousness around one male boss who was very critical. He told of his long history of both feeling dominated by men and feeling emasculated, going back to his father, who was an alcoholic and very harsh and critical. Walter spent a lot of time as a kid, and as an adult, trying to be perfect to avoid criticism.

Some of this talk happened before the session and some during the session. By the time I had reached the upper body we had a lot of this information. When I felt into his ribs on the upper back, he was very tense. I felt the same kind of tension in his anterior ribs in the chest. The energetic signature I felt in these tissues had the quality of working very hard to be perfect. He had to be constantly on guard, and that was easy to feel in the bones. There was a lot of protection and guarding in his tissues. He was holding himself tight, as if there was no room for error. And of course that would make him tense and tight.

Walter was aware of this. He said, "I spend so much time trying not to be criticized, trying to be perfect. I have had so much fear and shame about this."

I was very clear that I had to avoid any criticism of him to avoid triggering his old pattern, which would tend to push him to work even harder to be perfect. This can translate into wanting to be a perfect patient and to receive a session perfectly, rather than just let it happen. I wanted to support the positive parts of him, verbally, energetically

and with the Zero Balancing, and not be negative in any way. I didn't even want to try to get rid of the negative. I wanted to amplify the good parts of him rather than deal with the negative parts. I could do this both with my words and also with the quality of my touch.

My touches were all meant to be gifts to him. I made the touch feel as good as I knew how. I wanted to connect to his core. I wanted to find the new, fresh shoots of growth, and tend and support them. I was not trying to get rid of the "bad" or held parts of him but to support and amplify the good vibrations, the good feelings and the good energy.

Walter's body soaked this up like a sponge. I could feel major shifts in his body and his energy. His breathing deepened. The tissues relaxed. He had many more working signs including rapid eyelid flutter with his eyes closed, borborygmus, and slight vibrations of the head, all of which are signs of major change in the person.

He loved it. He felt much more connected, supported, positive and relaxed by the end, with a better understanding of where some of his fear was coming from. He felt so much better about himself. He was able to talk with humor and joy, and looked nothing like the slightly wild person who had come in.

In this case, deciding to support the positive aspects of Walter, rather than to try to remove or alter "negative" aspects, was working outside his pattern. Doing the same Zero Balancing session, but with a very different quality of touch and with a very different intent, countered his long-established pattern of self-perceived negativity and the resulting efforts to be perfect. I had started from a place where Walter was already good and healthy, and I built on that, with the idea that the freedom he gained in his body and his energy would generalize to other parts of his life.

Another case shows another aspect of amplifying the wellness with a client. Sometimes I talk in Zero Balancing about "tolerating" a feeling. When clients first hear the word, they usually don't know what I mean by it. Let me give you an example. In order to learn to ski, and to be a good skier, you need to be able to lean forward, down the hill. This puts your weight on the front of your skis and is what gives you control over the skis. The problem with this is it is very scary when you are first learning.

When I first started skiing, I thought, "Why would I want to lean *down* the hill? I could fall doing that. I would much rather lean back where if I fall it will be a short fall and I won't get hurt." The problem is that leaning back is exactly what will cause you to fall. So, you have to learn to tolerate the fear that comes with leaning forward in order to become a good skier. You learn that you can have the fear, tolerate that feeling and do what you need to do.

Sometimes in energy work the same principle applies. You have to learn to tolerate an unpleasant feeling that will change into a pleasant feeling if you stay with it long enough; or, you have to learn to tolerate something that feels so good you can barely stand it.

Vicky's frame from the start was to amplify her current expansion and maintain it. We were in the third day of an advanced ZB class, and she was already feeling wonderful and freshly expanded. She wanted to help that movement deepen and keep it going. This is the same idea we talked about in the last chapter on wellness, with Walter. In that case the client had a lot of difficult symptoms going on, but rather than focus on those symptoms we worked "beneath the pain" to find the wellness in the person and amplify that. In this case Vicky was feeling good to begin with, so it was easy to find the vibration of wellness or

happiness. My job was to help her expand that feeling in order to feel even better.

So we had a clear frame of what she wanted. Then, right before we started the session a surprising thing happened. She said to me, "I am nervous." I asked what she was nervous about, and she said, "What if it works?" What would her life be like if she had expansion all the time? She suddenly had a big fear of what she would be like and what she would do if she felt this good all the time.

There's another healing principle buried in this statement. How do we deal with doing well? How do we manage things when we feel good, when our efforts to change something are successful? It seems like this should be a piece of cake – that just feeling good should solve all our problems.

But it turns out things are not quite that easy. It is actually very common to have difficulty accepting the good in our lives. Some people feel guilty and wonder why they should have such a good life. Some people put more pressure on themselves to be more productive or contribute more to the community. Sometimes they have to deal with others' jealousy. Sometimes it is all so new and unusual that it just feels awkward.

This can bring unexpected difficulties. Feeling really good brings a greater flow of energy through the body. Being able to tolerate that greater charge in your body is not that easy. Sometimes it is almost more than one can bear.

On the lower half of Vicky's body – the first half of the session – all the places I touched and balanced felt good to her and to me. Her energetic field felt light and vibrant right from the start. In this session it wasn't so much about freeing up held tension as it was about getting in touch with the pleasant energy (the wellness), and increasing it by holding ZB fulcrums while in contact with the healthy energetic field.

As we went along she gradually started shaking a lot. Her whole body was shaking some, but her shoulders were shaking so much that she was having trouble getting a deep breath. I have learned that this shaking frequently means an excess charge of energy. The person's energy is building up more than she can easily integrate. There is more and more energy, yet the structure is still resisting some of the movement, like water building up behind a dam. This can make for a lot of tension, and it doesn't always feel comfortable to the person.

In my own personal work, often when I start to take deeper breaths it is painful or uncomfortable until I break through and the breath breathes me. It becomes natural and easy and then the tension is gone, and then I feel great. It's like clearing out the pipes or literally expanding the tissues and the vessels so they can carry more current. But at first it feels as if my body can't expand enough to allow the greater energy to move.

This was happening to Vicky. She had to be able to tolerate this unusual experience in order to move through it and get to a higher charge and a much more positive experience. At this point her eyes were closed. The first thing I had her do was open her eyes. I learned from one of my teachers, a psychotherapist in Argentina named Jorge Carballo, that the eyes are very important in energy work, and working with the eyes is a great way to discharge excess energy.

This made a big difference to her right away. Opening her eyes helped her calm down and feel less tense, less shaky and more able to breathe. She began to feel more pleasure in the energy buildup.

When I got to the upper half of her body, some of the same resistance was still there, but only about half of what it had been before. She was still shaking but not as much. She felt tension but also a lot of pleasure.

As we freed up the tension with the ZB, the shaking stopped and her breathing got more deep and regular. And then, suddenly, she was through that part of the session where there was resistance to the new energy. She had been able to stay with her feelings without stopping the process and without withdrawing her awareness. The tension left, and she began to feel totally good. The energy charge in her body was large. In fact, she felt super-charged. And she was completely okay with it. There was no more fear about "what if it works." She felt excited, alive, and vibrant.

When she got off the table she was lit up and looked bright and shiny. She felt a huge need to move. We often have people walk a bit after a ZB session to integrate the changes in their body and their movement. Vicky didn't just walk, she skipped across the deck at a very fast pace. The other students watching were amazed as this blur went racing by them. She ran to the ocean and ran up and down about one hundred steps several times, she felt so much energy.

Vicky continued to feel wonderful and look very bright, for the rest of the class and after. Because she was able to tolerate a very strong feeling that wasn't entirely comfortable she was able to move through it to a place of feeling wonderful. Just as a follow-up, I emailed my write-up of that session to Vicky a year later. She wrote back:

As I read I remembered the experience. I don't remember it as being uncomfortable... I felt completely safe to let the energy roll through... I remember I couldn't stop it until you suggested I open my eyes... it was a fascinating feeling... that energy rolling through... and... what I appreciated was feeling safe enough to let it roll through... to be with that amazing energy...

And yes... the skipping on the deck and the running up and down that beach path in my bare feet... I was so very full of energy... had to find an outlet... and I reiterate... it wasn't a bad feeling... quite the contrary... it was a super interesting and fascinating feeling... the ZB seemed to have opened something and the energy didn't know what to do with itself... or... maybe more plausibly... it was thrilled to finally be free and galloping around.

I remember how free I felt... how shiningly free (not a real word but it seems appropriate) and spacious and expanded... spacious... I think spacious is a good way to describe it... I felt so clear and so spacious and so grounded at the same time... really cool... it was a great space. It is a great space.

And, thank you for capturing it in words... it helped me remember back.... thank you for holding that space for me... that space that allowed me to expand into luscious spaciousness... clear, clear spaciousness.... and... as I write this... I sit taller... my eyes are shining... and I remember... I am that... expansive... and we can be that for one another and the world... expansive and clear and just that!

Thank you! and thank you ZB for helping each of us to see and be what we are.

V.

Chapter 13
Caring, Compassion, and Containment

Zero Balancing, and in fact all bodywork and much of medicine, involves taking care of the patient. Clearly the medical aspects are very important, but just as important are the emotional aspects. As I noted earlier, Michael Balint, a UK psychiatrist, was one of the groundbreaking physicians who emphasized the importance of psychologically-oriented techniques in medical practice. He said, years ago, "If doctors in their practice did not respond to and work with the psychological implications of what was happening in their patients, it was a major missed therapeutic opportunity." (Vaillant, 1997)

One of the often overlooked but crucial issues is the question of being taken care of. For many people it is difficult to let themselves be taken care of, even to the point of feeling deep shame or vulnerability. For some it brings up early childhood experiences of being cared for, or not being cared for. This issue is often tinged with feelings of fear or anger, as well as shame. The case below is an example of how good body work (in this case Zero Balancing), done with attention and caring, can help to ease or even resolve these feelings.

Georgia is a bodyworker in her thirties, familiar with ZB both as a receiver and a giver. She is a strong and independent woman. This particular session, she came in very upset. She was nearly in tears. She showed me her nose where she had been bitten by a dog on a home visit to a patient's house. It was a fairly bad bite though it had happened ten days before and by the time of this session had mostly healed. She was traumatized that it had happened. Plus, she was due to get married in less than two months and was upset that she would have a scar from it.

As we talked before the session, Georgia mentioned, in a mild voice, her rage. She was feeling the rage and feeling ashamed. She was worried that her rage made her unacceptable to her friends, colleagues and teachers in the Zero Balancing community.

She was worried that because she felt this rage, people in the community would think she was not good enough to be in ZB. She had resisted coming to me for ZB partly for that reason; her fear that I wouldn't be able to accept these feelings in her.

I reassured her that the community and I would urge her to allow her rage. (Though I also mentioned that one thing the ZB community doesn't always do so well is deal with anger. There sometimes seems to be an unspoken norm that you are "supposed" to feel good. So it made sense she would be afraid of her feelings being unwelcome.)

We processed her rage for a while. This included her rage at the woman patient, at the dog, at the people who took her to the hospital and even at herself for letting the dog bite her. Then we traced these feelings back to her mother, who had been negligent with her. This was a major source of her rage. After helping her clarify that this woman was different from her mother, I asked her where in her body she felt the rage. She pointed to her back ribs on the right side along the scapula, and to her neck.

We started the ZB session and the lower half was useful, but didn't feel totally engaged. We were still talking about her anger and what she could do about it. When I got to Georgia's upper back, her posterior right ribs were very sore and very held. These ribs were tight, hard and almost swollen. The energetic vibration I could read was anger and extreme holding. This holding felt as if it had been there for such a long time there was a deadness in the tissues. I had her bring her attention to those ribs, and as she did so she experienced the soreness. As the soreness subsided she discovered how good it felt to be touched there. I encouraged her to keep feeling that goodness.

At one point I asked her, "How does it feel it be taken care of in a good way, by someone who cares about you and won't be negligent?" She immediately burst into tears and sobbed for a minute or two. She was touched, and she felt met in a way she had wanted her whole life.

The depth of her wanting, and holding onto that wanting all of her life, had taken a big toll on her. She had been alone with the feeling and too vulnerable and ashamed to ask for the kind of caring she wanted. It was hard to let herself know what she wanted and how badly she wanted it. I think some of Georgia's independence came

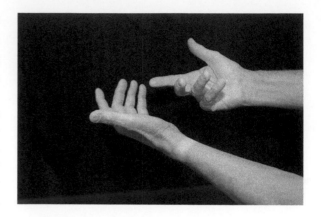

Fig. 13.1

The caring hands of Dr Fritz Smith.

(Photo: Giovanni Pescetto.)

from not being willing to let others take care of her, and perhaps not trusting that anyone would be able to take care of her. The change in her when she allowed herself to feel cared for was dramatic. She relaxed. She felt relieved and peaceful. She was okay to be herself.

After the tears I asked her how she was feeling. She said, "So much better, even good." Her ribs were considerably looser, with at least a 50% improvement. I did some more work on the ribs, and also on her neck and head. I still had her check into her body, regularly, to see what she felt. By the end of the session Georgia was feeling very good. She was less angry and more in contact with her core self. From that place she could take much better care of herself.

I did the closing fulcrums, which we do at the end of ZB sessions to help integrate all the change that has happened. After the session we talked for five to ten minutes about what she could do to deal with her anger. I suggested she could write for 15 minutes without stopping ("I am angry about..."). She could hit the bed with a tennis racket. She could talk to the people involved, saying she was angry but in a normal voice rather than shouting.

She felt grateful for the session, the caring and the suggestions for homework. She was feeling more open and trusting by then, so she asked me if "getting married was stressful for everyone." This was a new topic that she brought up just at the end of our time together.

I told her that on the stress scale getting married is about equal to the stress of getting divorced or someone dying. It is considered very stressful. That helped her feel much better and more normal. So we ended on a good note, with her feeling met and good about being cared for. I told her I appreciated her courage in bringing all these things up and staying with the feelings. This also made her feel good and lessened her shame. By the end, she was smiling.

This is actually a common experience for people who have a hard time being cared for. In Part One, Chapter 5 (the session with Max), as I tuned in to what I was feeling in his body, I realized that because he didn't feel worthy, he was not able to let in love or help or caring. It was as if he didn't deserve it.

I said to him, "Let yourself accept the caring and the help. See if you can allow in the caring and the compassion I have for you." He immediately changed. His body visibly, physically let go, and he started crying intensely. Afterwards he felt met in a deep part of himself and also much less confused. He had less anxiety, and his body felt lighter and clearer.

There are many ways of touching and showing compassion and caring. In addition to receiving information with his hands, the practitioner can also input information. The same way an actor can convey so much non-verbally, with a look or a gesture, a ZBer can impart an experience non-verbally. The therapist's hands can communicate almost any feeling by varying the quality of the touch. I can touch in a way that helps the client feel safe, met, connected and held securely. Or with a different quality of touch I can communicate an energizing feeling, and the client will respond to it, sometimes consciously and sometimes unconsciously.

There are many fulcrums in ZB that illustrate this idea. One I love to use is a fulcrum directly to the face, held with compassion.

Danielle is a Zero Balancer. I was doing a swap with her, where I would work on her and then we would trade around and she would do a ZB session on me. This is both a great benefit for a student, receiving a ZB session from a more experienced ZBer, and also a great way to learn from each other.

Her frame was about having kept herself going at a fast pace for a long time without being able to stop and take a break. She had not been able to listen to herself and to her need to let down or be taken care of. She had kept up a façade of being okay, even though it was not what she was feeling.

As the session went along, I could feel in her body the effects of what she had talked about in her frame. I could clearly feel the tightness and the tiredness and the holding in her tissues. So my goal in the session was to let her drop into awareness of a deeper part of herself that she had not accessed recently. I wanted to help her let go of any need to *do* and just allow herself to *be*.

Near the end of the session I did the fulcrum I mention above, one I often do with people I know well. I started by placing my hands very lightly on both sides of her face. I had light contact but stayed solidly connected to Danielle's donkey and to herself, with empathy and compassion. This fulcrum often produces the feeling in the client of being held as a young child, being taken care of with love and the kind of caring you would want from your "good mother."

Danielle got very soft and quiet during this fulcrum. Her body got still, and she had many of the working signs that indicate an altered state of consciousness. She said later she felt met and held, and felt that she could let her worries and struggles go.

After the session, Danielle said the experience of the compassion fulcrum on her head was incredible and the most important part of the session for her. This was the point at which she had been most able to let go of her holding and be herself. When I saw her again, later in the week, she said that she had been able to let go of her façade maybe for the first time in her life. It was a good reminder that Zero Balancing is not usually about the strength or the amount of pressure in the fulcrum – it is about connection and presence, qualities that can make the touch so powerful.

Another example of the same idea is using my hands to create a safe, soothing and containing feeling for the client. In most ZB sessions the predominant issue is to help people who have held themselves too tightly to let go and allow themselves to feel more of their emotions and their bodily sensations. In some sessions, though, the opposite is true. Some people feel so much emotion that they feel overwhelmed and disorganized (dysregulated).

The following session illustrates how we can work with Zero Balancing to help that type of person. In this case, I was working with a young, female acupuncture student, Mary, who was new to Zero Balancing. It was the first day of an Introductory Zero Balancing Class. In a ZB class I often teach how to work with a part of the body, then demonstrate the work on one of the members of the class, and they then all go the tables and practice that fulcrum on one another.

This demonstration was a fulcrum on the feet, called the two-handed foot fulcrum, aimed at freeing up the energy in the tarsal bones.

In most classes this is a straightforward demonstration, which feels good to the receiver,

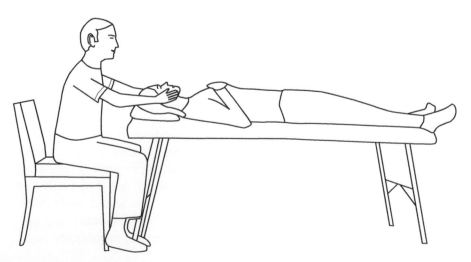

Fig. 13.2

A compassionate fulcrum held lightly on the side of the face.

but because it is early in the class, it often does not produce dramatic results. In this case, as I started to free up the energy in the bones of her feet, Mary felt an "energy" moving up her legs and then up her torso. And then a lot of feelings started coming up that were intense and scary to her. At one point she said the feelings were "very dark." She had a huge number of "working signs," including numerous deep breaths, rapid movements of her eyes and body shakes.

She was having intense sadness and tears but also a lot of fear. I don't remember if she said so or not, but it was clear to me that this was due to a history of abuse. (This was the first time I had met her, and as it was the first day of the class, I did not know her history when she got on the table.)

Mary was rapidly becoming dysregulated, which means she was overwhelmed by her feelings. She was having a hard time talking and didn't know what to do to stop the feelings. My job, which is usually to encourage clients to let their feelings happen, was to bring her back from

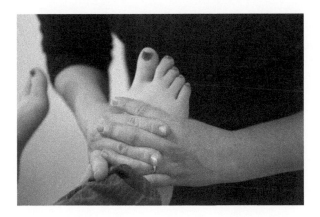

Fig. 13.3
Half moon vector to balance the tarsal bones in the foot.

(Photo: Della Watters; WattersWorks & Company.)

that overwhelming experience to be more aware of her present environment, where she was safe and with friends.

I asked her to "stay with me," which means I wanted her to keep her attention on me and her awareness in the room and in the present moment. I needed to keep saying this repeatedly, as she had a tendency to go back into the scary emotions. Keeping her awareness in the room helped her calm down and stay connected to herself, and to me and to the present moment. I also used a phrase common to this type of situation, "That was the past, this is now."

I did many fulcrums that are called "containing." The idea is to use a type of touch and a type of fulcrum that creates a feeling of clear boundaries and safety. This is like creating the feeling of swaddling a new baby so the child feels more contained and less overwhelmed by vulnerability. This is, in a way, the opposite of my work with Vicky in Part Two, Chapter 12, where I was trying to expand a positive experience. Here I wanted to help limit the experience so it wasn't too overwhelming.

After five to ten minutes of this containing touch, Mary was much calmer and very present. She was smiling and felt that the experience had been useful to her. She felt clearer and lighter and better.

So, freeing up something in her tarsal bones had unexpectedly freed up something in her whole system. It's common in a ZB session that fulcrums affect both the local area and the whole body, and almost every fulcrum has a global aspect, but in this case what got freed up was hard for her to deal with. With the right kind of verbal fulcrums and Zero Balancing fulcrums, I was able to help her calm down and make what could have been a disorganizing experience into a positive experience.

A person with a lot of working signs early on in the session is often a person with a history of trauma. The signs might indicate that the client's energy may move "out of her body" (dissociation) because the experience is too overwhelming. In the work with Danielle at the beginning of this chapter, I was able to give a feeling of compassion to a client by how I applied the fulcrum. Here I was able to use my touch to convey a presence and calmness that helped the client regulate herself.

Chapter 14
Boundaries

Setting clear boundaries is one of the first and most important duties of the practitioner of any therapeutic modality. Boundaries are necessary to create the trust needed to allow the client to relax and heal, and particularly to risk delving into personal issues. Poor boundaries can show up when a client is too easily influenced by others, feels invaded by others or causes others to feel invaded. This often leaves the client being out of touch with her own needs and desires.

One of the best tools for a Zero Balancer when working with a client with poor boundaries is to use *interface touch*, described in Part One, Chapter 5. Interface touch means keeping the practitioner's awareness where his hands meet the surface of the client, which helps to create a clear and safe boundary. During the whole of the session below, I kept my touch very strictly at interface, keeping a defined boundary between the client and myself.

This ZB session with Sheila, a female Zero Balancer from Canada in her early thirties, offers a good illustration of how important clear boundaries are and how difficult it can be to navigate them. Sheila attended a week-long advanced ZB class on Cape Cod. I had not met her before

that class. As the session went on, it became clear that I needed to help her develop much stronger boundaries, and I had to be aware to keep my own boundaries clear as well.

Near the end of the class I did a full Zero Balancing session with her. She was very upset from the outset of the session, but she was mostly trying to hide it or stop it. She was putting on a brave face, saying she didn't need a lot. The upset wasn't about what was happening in that moment. It was from some earlier time in her life. She was desperate for something, but too ashamed, too hopeless or too scared to feel and show what she really wanted. Sheila kept saying she was okay, but saying it with a grimace and looking away, or with the beginning of tears in her eyes. All these signals made it clear she wasn't okay and, in fact, needed a lot.

We talked some about what she wanted from the session. As we were doing that, I asked her more than once what was going on. She did tell me she had recently (within five months) come out of an abusive long-term relationship. She had suffered a great deal. My observation was that she had probably had a very hard time defending herself in the relationship. Her belief that she was unworthy led her to put up with that type of experience. It seemed to me that she desperately wanted someone to take care of her. These are all aspects of what I mean by poor boundaries.

Over and over Sheila would veer off or go into the details of her life and her past, but without mentioning the emotions that went along with the information. I kept directing her to pay attention to the sensations in her body rather than the information, as this would make it more experiential for her, and allow more change. This was very hard for her to do. She wasn't used to looking at her inner world, and said, "What do you mean?"

This is can be an important point in a session and requires what Sue Anne Piliero calls *psycho-education*. I told Sheila I wanted to help her learn how to pay attention to the sensations in her body, because this is where the information resides about what she is feeling and what she is wanting. It also would help keep her awareness in the present moment, as everything that she feels in her body is happening now. This allows more change to happen during the session, and helps a client afterwards make better, clearer decisions in her life.

Finally, I told Sheila that staying with the feelings in her body would help her build a stronger energy field and a stronger set of boundaries. This is the opposite of the dissociation we talk about in the chapter on trauma. Paying attention to your sensations helps you stay present and more organized.

I assured her that this process would allow her to listen to her inner self, to hear what she wanted and needed. This in turn would help her to feel less lost or confused, and perhaps prevent her from letting someone else tell her what she needed or wanted. It would help her hear what her body wanted, not just her mind. And it could

create a clear boundary between what she wanted and what others wanted.

I slowly persisted in helping her stay with her sensations. I asked her to close her eyes, to go inside and see what she noticed in her body. Whenever she would tell me she was "fine," I would say, "Keep checking into your body. What do you feel inside?"

As Sheila kept paying attention to what she felt inside, she began to feel more emotions and then to have a lot of tears. Sadness came up, both from the recent relationship and from childhood. The feelings she had been avoiding were allowed to surface.

We talked about those parts of her life as we did the session. Often as feelings came up, she would still want to escape from acknowledging them. She would tend to leave her body, which is to say, her awareness would leave her physical sensations, and her energy field would get more diffuse and less present.

When she tried to avoid her feelings, I could tell that she was less present. It would be as if we were walking along on a clear day with a long view of the sky, and all of a sudden the fog rolled in. Everything about her would get more vague. Her eyes would get cloudy. Her speech would get quiet and hard to understand, and the energetic sensations I felt from her body would become diffuse and vague.

At those times I would always ask her to bring her awareness back to her body, and the fog would lift. She would be present, and she could feel whatever was happening inside of her and in the room. Her voice and eyes would change, and the energetic feeling in her tissues would be more present as well.

I kept her in touch with her own experience of herself as much as I could during that whole session. I kept asking her over and over again to "listen to what you feel inside." And, as I said, I kept my touch at interface to make sure I maintained a clear boundary. This was necessary for her to feel safe enough to let herself explore her feelings.

The session took quite a while, as we kept stopping to help Sheila stay in touch with her experience. She was very sad for a lot of that time, but by the end she was feeling good. She felt "cleansed, refreshed, relieved and cared about." She felt like I was one of the first people in her life who really cared about her. Sheila felt that this was one of the first times in her life she had really been in touch with her wants and needs.

I suggested some homework for her after the session, which was to keep paying attention to her inner experience. I suggested exercises she could do in order to feel a clearer, stronger boundary, and also to keep from giving herself up in relationships. I talked with her about the importance of boundaries, which I think she had never had.

I told her "Whenever you feel lost or not sure what to do or not sure what you feel, go into your body and listen." This became our mantra. Afterwards she gave me a card with the phrase, "what do you feel inside."

We talked about how staying in touch with your body helps you create and maintain those boundaries. At one point she said to me, "You have very good boundaries," both appreciating that fact and also sounding a little wistful that I wouldn't give in and merge with her in the way she thought she wanted. I said "YEP! I have very, very, very good boundaries," acknowledging

the fact but also making it clear that nothing was happening between us outside the session. I cared for her, but as a way of helping her, not anything beyond that.

This was a particularly satisfying session for many reasons. The work I did both with my hands and with the relationship was high quality. The session helped Sheila go to a deep and important place for her, yet without engendering any kind of dependence. Quite the reverse, it strongly supported her independence and her ability to take care of herself, and to develop a healthier and happier approach to life.

Also, this session resulted in one of the greatest amounts of change in a person, in one session, that I have ever seen. She was lost when she arrived and found when she left. I don't know what has happened to her since, but she came in on a course that could have been extremely negative for her life and left on a course to a better life. This was gratifying, both for her and for me.

Finally, it felt good to let myself care for someone as much as I did during that session. I think at times, especially earlier in my professional life, I thought I was supposed to be detached. If I did feel something for a client, I would keep it to myself and keep it out of the treatment situation. I have since learned, from my work with Accelerated Experiential Dynamic Psychotherapy (AEDP), that it's okay, and actually good practice, to let myself care for my clients and be impacted by them, and to judiciously share with them some of that impact. In this case, my caring, along with clearly maintaining my boundaries, was a part of what allowed Sheila to make such an important change.

Chapter 15
Feeling Stuck

What is most interesting about the next session is that I didn't actually do any Zero Balancing. The whole session was devoted to talking to the client about what she was feeling, and this alone made a huge change for her.

Paula taught art and theater at a local college. She came in with serious trauma from a terrible car accident a few years earlier. I had worked with her one year earlier, with both acupuncture and Zero Balancing, which had helped her to get over the main physical effects of the accident at that time.

On this day, she came in saying, "My brain has started moving since the trauma, but my body has not. My body is still stuck. My body won't let go and my breathing is very bad from asthma. I am retaining fluids. I am exhausted all the time. My sleep is terrible, with 3–6 hours on a good night. My mind is going all night long. I get cramps and feel too hot."

She added "I've changed my diet a lot to less gluten, no dairy, no meat. I am eating only organic now, partly to help with my asthma. This has helped some but not much." The only positive thing she mentioned was that "my anxiety and anger are less than they were before."

I treated Paula with acupuncture for the first three sessions and all was unremarkable. There was not much change in any of her complaints from these sessions.

When she came in for her fourth session, my plan was to do some Zero Balancing, to see if that would make a bigger change for her. I asked right at the start how she was doing and she said, "Okay," but without much conviction. She really didn't want to make much contact or go into her feelings. She gave no further information. This left me feeling discouraged and also feeling how hard it was to make significant contact with her.

I asked for more information, and she said, "After the last treatment I got a terrible migraine the next day and didn't sleep well for two nights." I felt even more discouraged. I actually had a strong desire to give up and tell her we weren't making any progress and there was no point in continuing. Partly that was true, but partly I just wanted to be rid of this problem that wasn't getting any better.

Rather than doing that, however, I decided to get more assertive with my questions and my connection. I put down my notes, leaned forward and asked Paula to pay attention to her body and see what she felt. She said she was very good at helping other people to do that but didn't know how to do it with herself. She was "somewhat reluctant" to check into herself. She said she "wasn't able to feel connected to life," and if she did pay attention to her own experience she felt "vulnerable." We talked about the price she had to pay for not paying attention to her sensations, including not being able to feel her positive feelings.

Despite her reticence she closed her eyes and began to notice what she felt in her body. The first thing she said was she felt "sludge" in her chest, which was "dark and not moving." I asked her to stay with it. I wanted her to keep her attention in her body, being curious, non-judgmental and not trying to change anything. She talked about how she never does this for herself. It was a little hard for her, but she was gradually able to do it. At first she didn't feel much change in her chest, and she felt more pain in her inner scapula area and right shoulder, but as she kept paying attention finally the sludge began to lessen and her breathing got a little easier.

At one point Paula asked me why we were doing this since we had never done this before. I said things weren't changing, and we needed to take a different approach and see if we could get more to happen. She agreed with that.

As she kept paying attention, she felt more change. The sludge got less. Then she was quiet for a long time. I was wondering what she was feeling and then I noticed that I was beginning to feel sad. I realized I was resonating with her and asked her, "What are you feeling?" At first she said, "Not very much." I said, "I am beginning to feel sad. Are you feeling any of that?" She finally acknowledged that she was feeling sad. And slowly some tears started. After that there were a lot more tears, and she said, "The dam has burst."

After Paula cried for a while, I asked how she felt and she said, "Not good. I feel too vulnerable." I again asked her to locate that vulnerability in her body, if she could. As she did that, she felt the sludge go deeper inside, almost as if hiding. We talked about how she was trying to get rid of the sludge. I wanted her to feel and acknowledge the sludge and appreciate it for all it had been doing for her. Rather than bury these feelings and attempt to get rid of the vulnerability, I wanted her to integrate and transform these feelings.

She suddenly said, "I have a huge armor around me. I have for a long time because I never know what is going to happen. This is what keeps me from feeling vulnerable all the time." I suggested she might try a different kind of armor that could be put up or down as needed. And maybe that armor could be a little less thick.

We played with that idea for a bit and Paula began to feel more open. She started talking about how people she knows had transformed through work with Zero Balancing and acupuncture. She cried a lot more, and it was clear she wanted that for herself.

By the end of the session Paula felt much more relaxed and calm. She said, "This is huge." The dam had burst and after that the sludge was gone. She no longer felt stuck. I appreciated her for being able and willing to go deeply into her feelings, and I asked her what it was like to do that. She said it was very hard but very good and she wanted to do more. We both agreed this was what was necessary for her to move forward.

At the very end of the session she asked, "How it is for you to work with someone who is stuck and isn't moving?" I said, "It is very hard and tiring and even boring at times, but when you are changing like this I feel energized and not tired or bored at all. I feel good about what I have done and what you have done and what we did together. This kind of process makes me feel happy for you and alive in me."

She asked what she could do at home on her own. I asked her to check in to what she feels in her body 10–20 minutes a day without trying to change anything. I asked her to be friendly towards whatever she felt and watch and see what happens.

It was beautiful for me to see how much change was possible by applying these healing principles to connect with Paula verbally, just as I would with Zero Balancing. We kept at interface the whole time. I kept in very good contact with her during the session. We stayed with what she felt in her body. We stayed in the moment-to-moment experience and didn't drift too much into her story or why she felt what she felt. It's rare that I spend the whole time with someone talking without adding bodywork, but in this case it was necessary and the results were special.

Chapter 16
Overcoming Abandonment

One of my newer practices in ZB is to encourage the clients to say more about what they want, not only before the session but also during the session. If they want more pressure or less pressure, or to move the fulcrum a little left or right, or to check out an area of the body that I haven't worked on, I want to know that information. I have learned many times that they have access to feelings and information that I don't have. So I am happy to listen to their directions and try things out. If their suggestions don't accomplish very much, I can always move on and haven't lost anything.

In this session I let Fred direct the session to a large degree, and it turned out to be important for him and his session, but also for me in my learning. Fred is a man in his sixties. He works as an administrator. He is a big man with a dense body and a big heart. He is a dedicated supporter of other people. He's very generous with his time and with himself, and he is frequently smiling and engaging.

Near the end of a five-day class, I gave him a ZB session in the presence of four or five other ZB students. The class had been expansive and had involved personal growth work and openings

for a number of people, and Fred was willing to look at his own personal issues. He said he had experienced a lot of abandonment in his life and was longing for a deep connection. So the question was, could we find a connection through the touch of Zero Balancing that would allow him to feel met, held and loved? If so, my supposition was that this would have some carry over to how he felt in the rest of his life.

As I started the ZB session, I found that Fred was holding a lot of tension. The lower bodywork went well enough, but without major change. The tension was easing somewhat as we went along, but I hadn't been able to find that deep connection that he and I were searching for.

The upper body of a client is often a good place to help him connect to his own heart. A particularly good place to do that work is on the sternum. The sternum is thought of in ZB as the bony manifestation of the energy of the heart. As connection was the issue we were working with in this, I wanted to pay particular attention to Fred's sternum.

I put my hand on Fred's sternum and held it there a long while. Initially I wanted to explore what tensions and feelings were being held there

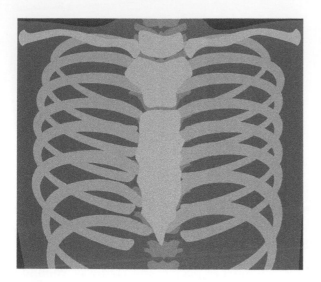

Fig. 16.1

The sternum, manubrium, clavicle and rib cage.

(Photo: Shutterstock.)

and also to see if this was a good place to connect with Fred. I felt a good connection through his sternum and thought it was going well, but he wanted more and asked me to press harder. I did press harder and that felt even better to me, but he still felt it wasn't enough to help him overcome his feelings of loneliness and abandonment. So I pressed as hard as I could with my one hand on top of his sternum, and used one hand to lift up underneath his body, with as much pressure as I could bring.

Fred's need to feel connected and to feel that he wouldn't be abandoned was very strong. He needed to feel a deep connection and to have it last a long time, to undo the feeling of having been left alone earlier in his life. I asked one of the students who was observing the session to put her hands on top of mine. She pushed hard and this added another layer of pressure to

the fulcrum through the sternum. The last layer came when Fred put his hands on top of the student's and mine and added his own pressure. We now had five hands on top of his sternum and my one hand pushing up from beneath, all pushing strongly. Finally, Fred began to feel the depth and quality of connection he wanted. He felt met. He could let go. This brought huge sobs as he grieved the lack of love and connection he had felt most of his life.

We all held that pressure and that connection for as long as Fred wanted. I wanted him to feel loved and held and met and that we were not leaving him. He stayed with this strong contact for a long time. He cried a lot. Gradually he began to feel more open and more relaxed. He stopped crying.

Finally, at his direction, we all let go. He looked and felt relieved, at ease, soft and grateful. Grateful that he felt better and grateful that we had stayed with him a long time and had not abandoned him. It was a beautiful experience for us all and came about because Fred was willing to say clearly what he wanted, and I was willing and able to follow him and to listen deeply to his needs.

The change in his body matched what he was saying. The tension was much relieved. His whole system felt connected and integrated. The sternum felt softer and more malleable. The other bones in his body were also softer and more accessible. His energy field went from being dense and tense to light and almost airy. A deep need had been met through the bodywork and through our energetic and emotional support and connection. As I watched him move around the room he looked very light, almost as floating, and with a distinct glow about him.

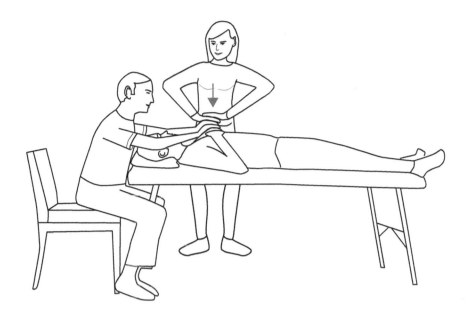

Fig. 16.2
Male client receiving pressure to his sternum and heart with six hands.

I think it was important for Fred to be able to control the depth of the touch and connection. It was also important to let him hold that connection for as long as he wanted. Both of those were important antidotes to his sense of abandonment. And for me, it was a lesson in trusting the client's awareness of his own needs and wants. This made a big difference in the session, and I've used that lesson a lot since then.

Chapter 17
Dealing with Anger

Anger is a difficult emotion for many people. It's hard when someone feels angry and doesn't know whether to express it, or how to express it. It's also hard when the person doesn't express anger right away, as it tends to build up as tension in the body and affect moods and behavior.

In addition, people are not so good at receiving anger, sometimes getting angry back or judging the other person for being out of control or overly sensitive. Another common response is to get defensive or turn away.

All of this is even more true in a health care setting, where there is often a clear power differential between the client and the practitioner. The following case is an example of anger felt and expressed by the client, and heard and received by the practitioner, in a way that led to both parties feeling good about the process, the outcome and each other.

During an advanced Zero Balancing class, I did a demonstration with Theresa on how to work on the tibia (shins) with Zero Balancing. Theresa is a long-time bodyworker and certified Zero Balancer, around 50 years old. She tends to be forthright about her thoughts and feelings and is a valuable member of any class she is in.

In the demonstration the fulcrum worked well, and she had a big experience from the fulcrum. There was a lot of change both in the bones of her shins and also a lot of energetic expansion overall. She felt good after the demonstration, even though it had only been five minutes of work.

We had a nice connection during the fulcrum that felt comfortable to us both. When she got off the table I went to hug her, which is common in a ZB class. In classes, this is often initiated by the client, and if I am unsure, I usually ask if the client wants a hug. In this case I didn't ask. I initiated the hug and it was one of those hugs that was not exactly met. It felt awkward and I wished I hadn't done it. Still, it didn't seem a big thing to me at the time.

Later that day we had a segment where I was working with a small group of people of which Theresa was a member. When Theresa's turn came up she didn't want to start doing ZB. She wanted to talk.

It took her a little while to get to what she wanted to say, and she started by saying vehemently that she was angry at me. I wasn't sure at first why she was so angry. As she talked more, she said she was really angry about the hug and really angry at me and at men in general. She was also angry at herself for not listening to herself and for disrespecting her own wishes. "I didn't want to be hugged and I let you do it anyhow. It made me so mad." Her voice was loud and strong and directed right at me.

I think in many cases I might have been scared and backed away or gotten defensive. In this situation I was able to stay present and stay with her and hear what she was saying. I asked her to say more about this, which she did, reiterating how angry she was. She was almost shaking as she was saying this, from the amount of anger she felt.

She said she wanted to do something and that she needed to move. I asked her, "What would you want to do." She said, "I want to knock you down and kick you." She said it with great vehemence and a lot of power. I wasn't afraid that she would really do it but I was on alert. I was aware of the amount of rage and the real desire to hit or kick.

I remained present. I didn't back away or get defensive. Nor did I go closer. I stood my ground and made eye contact with her. I invited her to bring in whatever feelings she had. I said, "I am not going anywhere." This also was important, as she knew she could express her anger fully and I was not going to go away.

She continued to want to hurt me. At one point I said to her, "I will not let you hurt me." I honestly don't know why I said that, but it turned out to be an important thing for her to hear. It allowed her to have all of her anger without the fear that she would actually hurt me. If anything, this statement seemed to help her calm down.

A bit later I said to her, "I can defend myself." Again this was soothing to her. She was slowly calming down. I held steady eye contact through most of this time. I also said, "I am sorry. I did not read the signals correctly."

The apology helped her lot. She said, "Yes, you did. I did want the hug, but I also didn't want it, so you did read it correctly, but there was this other part that didn't want to be forced or coerced."

By the time the conversation was over, Theresa had settled down and things were much clearer between us. She appreciated that I had listened and apologized and not gone away. The anger was mostly gone. And we both felt we had gone through a major experience and had handled it well.

Later that day, during a break in the class, we had a chance to talk again and go over what had happened. We both felt clearer by that time. We had a long chat and some laughter. Though now I can't remember much of what we said we connected in a deep way. We both felt met deeply. And later still, we had a mutual, sweet and deep hug, really meeting and without any baggage.

At the conclusion of the class, she said that it was "a life-changing experience, which she was very grateful for." Two things helped create that experience. One was that Theresa allowed herself to be angry and stood up for herself, to a male authority figure. Second, the person with whom she was angry was not defensive. I did not go away from her, did not abandon her, did not get angry at her in return, did not punish her in any way and, in fact, appreciated her for expressing herself so clearly and strongly. Both of us came out of the experience feeling clearer stronger and more connected to ourselves and each other.

Chapter 18
Resistance

Many clients come in for sessions saying that they feel tired or blah or down. They may say they have no energy or they have no motivation and don't feel like doing anything. Occasionally this can be due to significant illness or depression, but often it's due to the client repressing strong emotions that he doesn't wish to feel – grief, sadness, anger, fear or many other feelings. The content doesn't matter so much. What matters is that in order to avoid feeling the full impact of the emotions, he has deadened himself and his energy.

This is extremely common. So much so that my first question to a new client is often, "What do you feel in your body?" This almost invariably leads to emotions, which when expressed, free up the holding patterns in their body. Working with an awareness of emotions can free up the body, or working with the body can equally well free up the emotions.

Usually if I can help a client tune in to what he feels in his body, he can begin to feel his emotions. This is often uncomfortable at first, but can lead to relaxation, energy and positive feelings. A session with Frank, a student in his thirties, is a perfect illustration of this process. I did a demonstration Zero Balancing session in front of his class. This sometimes has a limiting quality,

as the person being worked on may feel nervous or awkward about being in front of a class of his peers. This had some effect in this session but also led to a deeper truth.

Frank came into the session saying he felt really tired. He felt no motivation and didn't want to do anything. He told me he wasn't usually like this, so he couldn't understand why he felt so unmotivated, but it had been going on for months.

The ZB session began slowly. As I did fulcrums on the lower body, Frank had some minor working signs of energy movement. He was getting deeper breaths but not deep breaths. He was getting rapid eye flutter but only some of the time. I could feel energy moving in his system, but I knew that with someone of his age, good health and a healthy body, there could be much more. As I was working I was wondering what could I do to help his energy build.

When I got to the upper body, I was working hard and still only getting a mild amount of change. I began using longer fulcrums with more pressure and more passes in the same area to see if that would help. Even with that I continued to feel frustrated, expecting more release than was happening.

There is a special fulcrum we do in ZB for the anterior ribs and lungs called the "inspiration fulcrum." The name is significant for two reasons. One, it refers to the inspiration of air into the lungs. Two, it refers to mental and emotional inspiration, which is generated by this fulcrum. In Chinese medicine the function of the lungs is to "bring in the inspiration of heaven," again with both meanings. This is often the perfect fulcrum for someone whose upper body is not opening fully and who also lacks motivation. This was a good match for Frank.

The fulcrum involves putting gentle pressure on the chest of the client as he exhales. The practitioner follows the ribs down during the exhalation, and when the client inhales the practitioner gives gentle resistance so the client has to work to breathe, which forces the lungs to expand more fully. I also ask the client to breathe into the upper part of the chest and the highest part of the lungs to fill the whole of the lungs with air.

This fulcrum made a bigger change in Frank than anything else we had done up to that point. Getting him to breathe up to the top of his lungs helped energize his whole system. Breathing more deeply is often a way to get more energy going, and Frank had more deep breaths and got both more relaxed and more energized.

I then went back to the upper ribs in his back and held the fulcrums longer, and there was more opening than before. The tension in his ribs lessened and this helped the energy build in his whole body. I could even feel a large change in the range of motion of his neck.

Nonetheless, I found myself thinking still more was possible. When we finished the session and he sat up, he was happy, to my surprise. He looked and felt lively and his eyes were brighter. He was smiling. He said, "I feel like myself for the first time in months." He felt energized. He felt ready to do things. So even though I knew more was possible, quite a lot had changed, and he felt much better.

When I asked him how the session had felt to him, he said, "At the beginning I was opening nicely and then on the upper body I began to resist you. I didn't want things to open any more. I was trying to stop it. So I actually felt less until you had me breathe way up in my chest. That really changed things and opened me up and I could feel more." This explanation of his experience matched my reading of the situation and helped me understand all that had been happening during the ZB session.

I asked him to pay attention to what he felt in his body at this moment. After he checked in to his sensations in his body, he said, "Anger." This was a surprise. I had not picked that up at all, and he was actually very angry. He felt good acknowledging the truth and speaking his anger. The opening from the Zero Balancing allowed him to finally let the brakes off and just say what he was feeling without holding back.

This in turn allowed him to feel even more relieved and freer and more energetic. He was behaving differently than he had at the beginning. It was clear his pattern of holding on to emotions and not speaking of them was a lot of what was causing his tiredness and lack of motivation. We learned this was especially true of his anger.

He had strong images of being really angry with someone. He was reluctant to go into details. He could see that he was still holding on some but couldn't stop altogether. Some things he was not willing to say in front of classmates. In the discussion with the class after the session, one of the students thought he had been sad, so I asked him in front of the class if he was sad, and he said "No – just the anger."

Later, after the class, he and I had a chance to talk further. There was no audience, and he said that he had also felt sad, but hadn't wanted to say it in the class. We talked about mourning the self and feeling sad for all the difficulty he had brought on himself by not sharing his feelings.

Then, he brought up fear, and said he had a lot of fear. I asked, "Fear of what?" And he said, "Fear of what people will think." He didn't want to talk about fear more than that. So, he was beginning to express his feelings but still had limits on what was okay for him to say.

He realized he needed to do work in this area. I gave him several suggestions of how he could work with these issues:

1. Suggestions for getting in touch with feelings. Pay attention to the feelings and sensations in his body. I suggested he spend some quiet time really noticing what was happening in his inner world. This would give him clues to what he was feeling earlier, and having that awareness would be the first step to helping things change.

2. Write down what he noticed. Once he was aware of what he was feeling, he could start to work with the feelings just by writing down what came to him. I often suggest to clients that they write for 15 minutes without stopping, writing down in a stream of consciousness whatever comes into their minds. He could start out writing, "I am angry at _____" and just go from there. The idea is to get deeper thoughts out so that the client is aware of them, and this helps the energy field move.

3. Talk more to people. Once he had become aware of his feelings and explored them a bit by writing them, he would be much more ready to express his feelings to other people. It could be the people he had feelings about, or others who could listen. Just the process of verbalizing his feelings would make a big difference, in behavior, in how he felt and in his body.

4. Get more ZB. Several more ZB sessions would help his system open and give him more access to his feelings. Sessions might reduce a lot of the armor that results from holding feelings in. That alone would help him feel better and also help him be more able to deal with his feelings with other people.

Frank left the workshop feeling very good and proud of himself for taking the risk to share his emotions. He also felt more energy and motivation. He was smiling and ready to do more work on himself.

To me, it is interesting to see what happens in the body when a person is unaware of, or avoiding, feelings. Feelings are an energetic vibration. An emotion that is too strong to be processed or accepted in the moment gets repressed and pushed out of awareness. If that vibration is not allowed to be freely felt and expressed, it gets ossified in the body. The physical body gets tighter, energy in the body gets lower, the emotion gets weaker and the motivation gets lost.

Basically Frank had been withdrawing and, in the process, isolating himself, and his body was getting tighter and less lively. The tighter he became, the less he wanted to share what he was feeling. This created a resistance to feeling anything at all. And when the resistance began to soften during the ZB, he felt more and expressed more and began to get his liveliness and motivation back.

This happens over and over again in all parts of our lives. Zero Balancing helps the process of

91

freeing up clients by identifying where the vibrations are held in the body. With gentle pressure into the held areas, especially the bones, these tight areas begin to loosen, and the client begins to feel more freedom of movement and emotions. The oft-stated message of this book is the correlation between mind and body, and how freeing the body frees the emotions and vice versa.

As I said in Chapter 4, in ZB we find that the deepest hurts, the emotions denied most strongly, end up causing significant holding in the bones. The holding literally causes the bones to change their quality. A whole bone can get dense or brittle or dull, or sometimes the whole skeleton will be affected in that way. Or one area within a bone can become dense like a knot in a branch. Gentle pressure to those held places within the bones, with ZB fulcrums, is enough to free up that held energy. This freed energy usually leads to the client feeling more emotions, but also to the repressed or denied energy being allowed to move and become available.

Chapter 19
Anxiety and Depression

One of the basic tenets of Zero Balancing is that if you balance the energy flow through the skeletal structure, you can positively influence the balance of the whole person: body, mind and spirit. One of the biggest questions for me when I began Zero Balancing was how effective bodywork would be with strong emotional states, particularly anxiety and depression. Over the years my personal experience with Zero Balancing has shown ZB to be very helpful to many people with these conditions, especially with anxiety and some forms of depression.

The research done by the Zero Balancing Touch Foundation in 2017 and 2018, cited in the introduction of this book and in Chapter 23, confirmed my clinical experience.

Research findings

The researchers found there was on average a 61% reduction in client anxiety (and also stress and tension) after one thirty-minute Zero Balancing session. Both the Zero Balancers and the clients were measured, with electrical sensors, on six different physiological scales. They also answered questionnaires about their states before and after the sessions. The objective physical measurements obtained from the sensors and the subjective replies to the questionnaires had the same findings. In comparison, a client lying on the table with no treatment had a 12% lessening of tension and stress.

(You can get more information on this study by visiting the website of the Zero Balancing Touch Foundation, zbtouch.org, and clicking on the Research tab.)

The following case is one example of how Zero Balancing can have a major impact on a client with significant anxiety and depression. Hillary was a woman in her forties who was new to Zero Balancing and acupuncture. She had a significant history of depression and anxiety. She came to see me soon after her mother's death. At the time, she felt a lot of fear and anxiety that her mother's death would push her into a depression that she would not be able to get out of. This was based in part on previous experiences with depression, but even more so on a free-floating fear of the mere possibility.

Hillary said she spent a lot of time and energy holding herself with a lot of control to keep from feeling too much and thus triggering further depression. I knew before I put my hands on her, from talking with her, that she had fears, but I had no idea how strong they were until I felt them in her body. The tissues felt almost knotted or twisted, as if they had been wrung out like a bathing suit or towel.

At the beginning I didn't know exactly what this knotted feeling meant. As we went along I understood that she was holding this tension and tightness on purpose, rather than unconsciously, as is the case with most people. To me, she seemed frantic at the thought that some feeling might get through and into her awareness. It was quite stunning.

Her goal for the ZB sessions was to find a way to relieve her feelings of grief and sadness without descending into depression. To help her achieve her goal I decided to go very slowly with the ZB and try to release one layer of tension at a time. I wanted to avoid her having too strong a surge of emotion that would push her over the edge. I also wanted to move slowly with the ZB to help her feel some control over the process.

The first full ZB session was pretty conservative, and it helped me evaluate how this strategy would work for her. The session went well and had a good outcome. Moving slowly enabled her to allow more emotions to emerge without feeling overwhelmed. She felt safe enough to cry, but never felt out of control. She felt much better afterward.

With that positive result in place, I was now free to continue with more ZB in that vein. In the second session, the Zero Balancing was most effective in her upper back and neck, especially the ribs in the upper back, which is where I had felt the most excess tension initially. The tension began to shift subtly right away. These tissues got less tense, and she felt, correspondingly, less fear and anxiety.

The lessening of tension brought some relief and good feelings, but shortly after that she began to feel a rise in her fear. This fear was different from just feeling more emotion. This was her fear that feeling any emotion would lead her into a serious depression.

I paused the ZB for a bit and talked with Hillary to reassure her that what was happening was normal, common and actually beneficial. *Verbal fulcrums* (see Chapter 11), talking and sharing suggestions and insights, play an important role in helping educate clients on how to move through what arises when the mind and body changes happen in ZB. I explained that freeing up held energy often leads to more emotions, but over time it can lead to less tension, less fear and more energy and well-being. She was relieved to hear that. She felt vulnerable but she was able to tolerate that feeling and let the session continue.

Freeing the tensions in a client's tissues or bones gives the person more ability to feel all of her emotions, both the pleasant ones and the unpleasant ones. She can often feel more pleasure but also sometimes more pain, both physically and emotionally. This can lead to contraction again unless it is addressed right in the moment. With Hillary it was crucial to address the rising fear immediately, and that helped to calm her and help her regulate her emotions. It was also crucial to keep moving slowly, a little bit at a time, so she wasn't overwhelmed. Hillary left the second session still feeling vulnerable but overall much better and less afraid, less anxious and not depressed.

Over time Hillary had less and less anxiety and depression. At each session she reported having felt better right away from the previous session. Her body became progressively less tense, in a much more normal range. She came in smiling for several sessions and reported feeling better, with much less depression and much less fear or anxiety.

We had one session where I pushed her, verbally, to express more of what she was feeling, and her anger at her mother arose. She cried strongly, the only time she had done that with me. Her fear had diminished to the point that she could let herself feel deeply and at the end of this session she again felt better.

This allowed me to point out to her that feeling a lot of emotion doesn't always lead to feeling worse, and to depression. In this case she felt better after having strong feelings, and I wanted to emphasize this to her, as evidence when facing these kind of situations in the future.

The experience of these sessions reinforced two ideas. First, the body doesn't lie. As we have seen over and over again, Bessel Van der Kolk's book title, *The Body Keeps the Score,* is true. The physical body's condition accurately reflects the emotional condition of the person. And, second, Zero Balancing can indeed be helpful for both anxiety and depression.

Chapter 20
Trauma and Zero Balancing

My experience has shown that bodywork in general, and Zero Balancing in particular, has a lot to offer to clients with a significant history of trauma. This is echoed in the writing of a number of psychiatrists and psychologists who work with trauma patients. Many are coming to the conclusion that working with the body is an important element of therapy with these clients.

Working with clients with a history of trauma is very different from working with people who do not have that history. There are numerous good books on this subject. (Especially good are *The Body Keeps the Score* by Bessel Van der Kolk and *Waking the Tiger* by Peter Levine.) I will not try to repeat that information here. My goal here is simply to explore my experiences doing Zero Balancing with this group of patients. It's worth noting at this point that most of these clients who I see with Zero Balancing are also working with excellent psychologists or psychiatrists.

In ZB we have tools and ways of watching the body's signals that help us identify clients who have these issues. There are a couple of key words that have particular meaning in Zero Balancing and that are useful to define as we talk about working with trauma. *Depletion* means a significant deficit of energy. This can come from a variety of causes. Many forms of stress and illness, including mental illness, as well as a history of trauma, can lead to major energetic deficiencies in people who have these problems.

A client I worked with years ago had serious trauma as a child. This included her parents putting out cigarettes on her skin and a list of other physical and psychological traumas. When I first went to work with Maria, I could not get her energetic field to be coherent. I remember saying that her energetic field felt like "wet tissue paper." It felt soggy and without form. As I tried to build the integrity and coherence of her field, it would collapse if I added one ounce too much pressure. Among other things, this led to Maria feeling weak, disorganized and extremely tired. She provided a clear example of how depletion from repeated traumatic episodes shows up in the body's energy field and tissues, as well as the psyche.

Dissociation occurs when the person cannot physically get away from a traumatic situation, so she leaves energetically. This creates a distinct feeling in the tissues. A body, or part of the body, where there is dissociation often feels cold and almost lifeless. I treated a friend who had had a severe biking accident, breaking her elbow in seven places. It took her a year to heal from the accident. I saw her the day after the accident and her right arm felt like cold, dead meat. There was very little aliveness or consciousness in the tissue.

With dissociation, the energetic field of the person becomes extremely diffuse, and this can lead to the person feeling unfocused, ungrounded and out of contact with the self and the environment. Depletion and dissociation are related because dissociation often leads to depletion. When a person leaves her body by dissociating, her energy automatically becomes weaker, thus depleted.

This group of people tends unconsciously to continue to be disconnected from bodily sensations long after the traumatic events, usually to avoid feeling the distress that stems from these events, and this leaves them feeling depleted over time. A common way this shows up early in a ZB session is when the client is having an excessive number of deep breaths, and a large amount of rapid eye flutters and body movements. As we have seen in other chapters, in the right amounts, these signals are positive working signs of a person being in a beneficial altered state of consciousness, but an excess amount of these same working signs can be an indicator of depletion, where the client is getting very low on energy and is staying unaware of his body. The client is unconsciously working to stay depleted, because when his energy field gets stronger he often starts to feel more difficult emotions.

Other common bodily signs of depletion or dissociation that we see in Zero Balancing are prolonged shallow breathing, very poor voice quality and a limp or languid body. All of these say to the Zero Balancer that the client is

beginning to lose energy and get less organized. This can occasionally happen in a ZB session if we hold the fulcrums too long or let the session go on too long.

ZB sessions with Mandy and Elaine can give a glimpse into how Zero Balancing can be beneficial to a client with a history of trauma and how those sessions might be different from a session for clients without trauma. Mandy is a 30-something-year-old female who had been receiving Zero Balancing for several months. It has generally been very beneficial to her. After a few treatments, she said, "Having these treatments is allowing me to have my core, which allows my feelings to come up. More feelings and more memories have come up." She was reporting this as a good event even though a lot of the feelings that came up for her were painful.

During her first ZB session Mandy said she was feeling "jagged, shaky, head wobbly, and with a big knot in my stomach." She felt "extremely tired and no energy." These feelings were quite intense. She said she felt "so awful I am not sure how I can endure it."

She began to describe the details of her memories and of her childhood. The traumas she endured involved being tortured and being held in a very painful way on her head. As a child she wished she were dead. It would have been a relief to be dead.

As she was talking about how she felt in the session, I asked her to pay attention to what she felt in her body and particularly to pay attention to the knot in her stomach. My job in ZB with this kind of client is to gradually help build her awareness of the present moment and of her physical body. This will help her feel more solid and grounded. It will also help her build a stronger energy field. She will slowly, over time, be able to tolerate her uncomfortable feelings more easily.

There are many ways to help a person develop more skill at keeping in touch with her physical body. We can ask her to pay attention to what she feels in her body, as I did with Mandy. Often this will not be easy for these clients, and we may need to take some time to educate them on how to feel what's happening and how to stay with what they do feel.

In this case, Mandy was able to comply with my request, and after she paid attention to her body for a while, I asked what she noticed. She said, "The sensation got easier in my gut, less shaky, with more energy movement." I asked her to stay with it, and she then continued to feel into the sensations in her body. She began to get sad and then to feel rage. I paused at this point of the session, as the feelings were getting so strong she was beginning to be dysregulated. The client may be overwhelmed by the feelings in this kind of situation, and it is something to be avoided when possible.

We discussed what had happened, and she said at first she had been afraid to feel in her body. She didn't really want to feel the "anxiety and then the fear and the feeling of wanting to be dead." To her, feeling anxious was almost the same as feeling she was going to die. The anxiety was tied to the abuse, and when she felt that abuse she wanted to die. And she was afraid that if she began to feel those feelings she wouldn't be able to get away from them.

We did some work to uncouple those two ideas. "Anxiety is not equal to death. You were scared of dying as a child but are not going to die here. You are safe here." All of this was to help her get in touch with her adult self and to see that she was actually safe in the moment. This did turn out to be helpful, and she began to calm down again.

After several ZB sessions Mandy had done a lot of work and had already made significant change in how she felt. We started the next ZB session on her lower body. She still had an excess of working signs, but all of the initial work in this session felt wonderful to her. This continued to be true when we got to the upper body and worked on the ribs in her upper back.

We both felt it was relaxing for her. Initially, I felt a lot of tension in her body, but as I held the fulcrums that tension lessened appreciably. She described the experience as "relaxing my armor." This was accompanied by a pleasant feeling of more energy in her body. Once she didn't have to spend so much energy protecting herself, she had much more energy overall. She felt "less heavy and less tired." This was evident to me in her body. The energetic feeling in her tissues under my hands got clearer, stronger and less heavy.

When I went to her head, she started to resist again and to protect herself. I could feel this immediately even though she didn't say anything. I could feel the tension in her whole upper body increase. So, we paused again and I asked her what she was noticing. She said, "Some of the trauma I suffered was on my head, so I always feel the need to protect my head." I thanked her for telling me. I wanted to help her feel she had control over what happened to her head, and that I would listen to her and we could move at a pace that was as comfortable to her as possible. And, that we would stop at any point if she wanted me to.

One of the keys to doing bodywork with people with a severe trauma history is to help them feel in control of what is happening. They need to know they can stop the session at any point if it doesn't feel right, or if they start to get overwhelmed, or if they just don't like it. Part of what makes something traumatic is that it is a bad experience and the person can't stop it and can't get away from it. It is important that the client feels safe enough to stop the session at any point.

We practiced several times where I gently held her head and I said to her, "Ask me to put your head down." She was very polite and she said, "Please put my head down." And I did, and she felt really good about being heard and listened to. Very shortly after she asked me to pick up her head again. Once the fear was gone, the feeling was pleasant to her. We did this a couple more times, and each time after she asked me to put her head down, she soon asked me to pick it up again. This helped her relax a lot, and she was able to have me do much of the work I often do on any client's head. And then she said, "That feels like enough." She had done a lot of good work that day and was feeling proud of herself and feeling good. She was glad to stop there.

After the session, when she sat up, she was not feeling shaky or tired or jagged any more. She was feeling energized and much more relaxed. We both realized how much energy she had been putting into holding onto that armor and keeping it in place. I said, "You were protecting against the kind of things that happened to you."

She said, "I am protecting against myself and against my own fears and feelings. I was very afraid that if I felt my feelings and felt the fear I would feel despair and go down a hole I could not get out of. This can get so bad and so horrible it might lead to death."

The bodywork with Zero Balancing, and simultaneously working verbally to help Mandy keep her awareness in her physical body and in the present, helped to lessen the effect of the trauma. The bodywork helped to free up the physical and energetic tensions. This allowed more of her feelings to come into her awareness and then helped her tolerate those feelings. The combination of the two types of work was powerful and healing for her.

There are many ways to help a person keep in touch with her physical body during a ZB session.

We can ask her to pay attention to what she feels in her body, as we saw here. Often this will not be easy for her, and we may need to take some time to educate her on how to feel what's happening and how to stay with that.

Another useful request is to ask her to keep her eyes open during the session and to observe what is around her. This helps to keep her awareness present in the room and avoids drifting and "spacing out," which leads to more depletion and often to more intense unpleasant feelings. Having her do exercises with her eyes is also helpful. Moving her eyes in a circle while keeping awareness on what she is seeing, or looking far away and then close up, also with awareness, helps her stay present.

Often in Zero Balancing we help to free up held energy, and we let the body sort out where that freed energy will go. We are following the client's lead. With trauma patients we are more likely to lead, to help them stay in tune with their bodies as much as they can tolerate. We may have to educate them as to why we are working in this particular way, even though sometimes they don't like it as much. They may like and be used to the feeling of being depleted or dissociated but we think it is not helpful to them. Often a typical ZB session will occur with no talking. However, with people who are getting depleted or dissociating, keeping up a conversation with them during the session helps hold their awareness in the room and in the present moment and helps keep their fields strong and intact.

As we saw earlier in Chapter 13, how we use our hands in ZB also affects the receiver. Shorter, possibly slightly painful, fulcrums are more tonifying and help to build energy and keep the client present in her body. Generally, shorter sessions are useful for people with trauma.

All of these techniques help the ZB sessions go well and help the client build a stronger energetic field. Many of these same techniques can be used at home by the client to continue and maintain the progress made during the session.

Another example of a session with a client with a trauma history is with Elaine, a 40-year-old medical doctor. She has received Zero Balancing sessions many times. She has a significant history of trauma, though we have never discussed the details.

In this session I noticed as soon as I put my hands on her shins at the beginning of the session that her energy field was fuzzy, not focused and not strong. As I discussed in the first part of this chapter, a diffuse field is common with people with trauma. This is a sign of dissociation where the client is not very present in her body.

Immediately I knew that I had to do a ZB session taking into account this history. That meant doing a shorter session, with short staccato fulcrums rather than holding fulcrums for long time. Fulcrums held a long time with this sort of client often encourage them to space out more. In contrast the rapid staccato fulcrums tend to build up the weak energy field and help the person be more present to the moment. I was also paying particular attention to bringing her awareness more into what she felt in her body, both by using a more physical touch and by talking with her during the session as necessary.

The torso is done near the beginning of most ZB sessions. As I moved to Elaine's torso, these same feelings of fuzziness, weakness, and dissociation were particularly pronounced in her lower right rib cage and right lumbar area.

When I am working with a client I often have a split level of attention. Part of my attention is focused on what I feel in my hands; partly on the working signs of the client and partly on the reactions in my body in response to the work with the client.

In this session, even though I had made a note of the dissociation and intended to do the kind of fulcrums I describe above, I suddenly noticed in the lumbar area that I had been spacing out – that my own awareness was out of touch with my body. My energy was getting unclear and my attention had drifted from her to a sort of daydreaming. I had lost interface without noticing.

One of the ways to help a client who is dissociating to stay present is to talk to them. So, when I become aware of this happening to me the first thing I do is check in with the client by asking what they are feeling. This has the dual benefit of giving the practitioner information about the state the client is in, and at the same time helping the client to become more present.

Usually they have energetically left their body and sometimes their energetic experience is so strong that it's easy for the practitioner to get lulled into a very similar state. If the practitioner allows this to continue the client usually will end up feeling weaker and less clear.

When dissociation is happening things cannot shift. Things are held in a sort of lockdown where no one is home to monitor how things are doing and how to respond. It's as if the person is on autopilot, like when you drive right by your exit on the highway. Even though you are fine to drive, your awareness is not really on what is happening around you.

This is a time in a Zero Balancing session when the practitioner needs to interrupt what is happening and help the person get more present to their bodily experience.

In this session, when I asked Elaine how she was feeling, she said she felt "spacy and mostly not present to my body and to what we are doing."

So I continued the conversation with Elaine, while continuing the ZB with the kind of fulcrums I describe above. She began to talk about how she loses presence in her life and when that began. A recent visit home had reminded her of the degree to which her parents were never present emotionally. She noticed how she was "likely to follow their lead" when she was with them, and to go unconscious herself, where her awareness would be in a sort of la-la land, rather than on what was right in front of her. Elaine received no reward for being present, either in her current life or as a child. She had no role model to show her how to stay present in her own body.

Once we both got clear on what was happening I asked Elaine if she was able to become more present to what she felt in her body. She was able to do this and it immediately caused her energy field to be more focused and clear. This allowed shifts in her body that had not been happening before. She could feel the effects as her body got more unified and organized and her awareness got clearer and stronger.

We worked together to hold her present for the rest of the session by helping her focus on what she felt in her body. As she paid attention to her inner state she began to have tears and to have more desire to talk.

She said one of her therapists had described her as a strong force but one that could easily be blown off her direction. I found that too. I found her very capable of being present, and yet, very inconsistent. She "checked out" frequently.

She talked about her parents never meeting her mentally or emotionally and how she deserved to be met. She said "I have spent much of my life wanting to get away from myself." She was sad for what she'd never had and sad for having taken so long to do the work to re-connect with her inner self.

I continued doing the ZB as we talked. By the end of the session she felt very met and touched. This was an important part of the process. For this client we want the inner changes of awareness to happen and for her body to change, but even more important is that she begins to be able to be present to the relationship. We want her to be able to be with another person and still stay connected to herself. We want her to have the experience of being met by another, in this case the ZBer, and to be able to tolerate that connection and intimacy without having to get away from herself or from me.

After this session she was much more able to do that and to be aware of the sensations in her body at the same time. She began to notice that the experience of being connected was, in fact, pleasurable. She felt grateful.

By opening up to the sensations in her body, being present to her feelings (meeting herself), and meeting me, she had opened up a place of aliveness and joy in herself.

Part Three

Body, Mind, and Spirit

Chapter 21
Unifying Body, Mind, and Spirit

It is a common experience for people to repress their feelings. This is usually because the feelings are painful initially, and most people don't want to feel that pain. Another common reason to hold on to emotions is to try to protect ourselves in an effort to feel safe. Many children experience shame, abuse or other negative consequences for saying their feelings out loud, and thus learn not to talk about them. This often leads to not being connected to their feelings and experience.

The truth is that this type of repression often leads to a deadening for the person, and she might have a hard time feeling her positive emotions as well as her negative emotions. This may show up as depression, anxiety, fatigue or a certain kind of numbness. When we help people become aware and tolerant of their feelings, they often experience a marked change in mood, energy and well-being. Even when the feelings aren't pleasant, they are real, and experiencing that reality opens the door to more positive change.

This section of the book looks at how a series of Zero Balancing sessions can affect a person over time, and also illustrates once again the often dramatic relationship between the mind and the body. This client's physical changes while receiving several Zero Balancing sessions were accompanied by profound changes in her emotions, and in her relationship to longstanding patterns in her life.

Nancy is a potter in her fifties who had come for ZB off and on over the years. As she had a history of Zero Balancing we often just started right into the bodywork without a lot of initial talking. In one early ZB session, we began with the typical ZB protocol, starting with a half moon vector and then working with the lower ribs and then the sacroiliac joint in the pelvis. The most striking thing about the beginning of the session was that I couldn't feel connected to her at all. I could easily feel the bones and ligaments and muscles, but I didn't feel Nancy – her thoughts and feelings – as I usually did with clients. As we went further into the session, I began to see that she was having a hard time connecting to herself. That is, she had limited awareness of her own body sensations and emotions. It seemed to me that she was actively avoiding these parts of herself.

I said to her, "It feels as if you have a hard time connecting to yourself. It feels as if you actually want to avoid connection and to avoid being in touch with yourself and others." She agreed, which surprised me, saying she didn't feel connected to herself and was very leery of connecting.

Having my impressions confirmed caused me to change how I was doing the Zero Balancing. I began holding the fulcrums for a longer time to allow space for her to feel what was happening inside. As I held the fulcrums longer, I began to feel more in touch with Nancy and her donkey, and thus in touch with her energy field. Once this began to happen I found I could hold the fulcrums in a way where I could allow and encourage her to connect to her own sensations more fully.

There is a stronger feeling in the tissues when a person is connecting to her own donkey. The energy field gets more vibrant and lively. The practitioner can easily feel this, and the client also knows she is in touch with her own being, which changes her experience and her body's response to the session.

As I did this ZB session, I paid special attention to places where I found more engagement with her and a stronger energetic response. I wanted that sensation to make an imprint on her nervous system. I wanted to help her lessen the fear of feeling connected by helping her experience her deep emotions more fully.

I held these long fulcrums with strong connection, and this became a powerful session. Once she tuned in and embraced her own feelings, Nancy had a lot of grief, pain and tears. Allowing herself to feel these difficult emotions allowed us to have a more free-flowing dialogue. She was aware how her desire to avoid connection was a way of protecting herself but was also very limiting. She began to express emotions and thoughts that had been hidden. She became aware of her strong feelings of wanting to protect herself.

As we worked further I felt a very young part of her. This part of her was nervous and fearful. There was almost a lack of maturity in her body, which showed up as soft and fuzzy edges in the tissues, without clear definition. We talked some about her early childhood and her relationship with her mother. She said how arbitrary her mother was and how she never knew what to expect and thus was constantly on alert. This explained a lot of her fears and her need to be vague and undefined, thus becoming less of a target for her mother's wrath.

By the end of the session she felt much calmer and much more in touch with all of herself, the painful parts, but also the alive and vital parts. Letting herself experience her grief and pain allowed her to let go of some of her old patterns of avoidance. She was more relaxed, as she didn't have to protect herself so much and she didn't have so much fear of expressing herself or feeling her own inner sensations.

This turned out to be an important session for Nancy. There were big changes in the tissues in her body and big changes in her being. By the time we finished the session, she looked and felt like a new person. She looked as if she had just come out of the womb, extremely young in a healthy way, fresh and alive. When I mentioned this to her she said she felt the same way, and as if she had "shed something."

This session is a perfect example of the benefit of going into the emotion and not avoiding it. The process produces much more presence, energy and aliveness. Fritz used to say, "The way OUT is THROUGH," meaning you need to tolerate what you're feeling to help change happen.

This session helped build my relationship with Nancy and helped our work go even deeper later, when she came in for what was originally a physical complaint. She came in after a hard fall down the stairs. She had caught herself on her hands and had bad breaks in both wrists, though the right was worse. The radius on her right had been displaced and slid down towards her palm. She made her living mostly with her pottery, and she had been out of work since the fall, with casts on both hands a lot of that time.

She had tried several other therapies before coming to see me. These therapies had been somewhat helpful. She was doing well enough to get back to work but was still very limited in what she could do. Along with the physical limitation and discomfort, she was feeling very distant from herself again, as in the earlier session above. She was not back to feeling like herself, though it had been five months since the fall. She also felt weakness, specifically in her abdomen.

I asked her to sit on the table and looked at her wrists and arms. I started evaluating the range of motion in her wrists – the quality of motion in flexion and extension, side-bending, and rotation. The range of motion on the right wrist was dramatically limited in several directions, with extension particularly restricted.

Then I examined her forearm. The radius and ulna, the two bones of the forearm, were way out of position, leaving her whole hand looking distorted. When I looked at her right elbow, internal and external rotation were both very limited. Her right shoulder and ribs on that side had limitations as well. So the whole of her right arm and right side was affected.

As I considered these findings, my first question to myself was where to start, with so many areas significantly out of balance. I decided to start on her right forearm rather than the typical ZB protocol of starting with the lower body. The feeling in those bones was so unusual that I suspected we needed to improve these bones to get much change anywhere else.

The bones were so soft and flexible that the image of Gumby, the cartoon character, came to mind. We talk in ZB about "bone-bending" and the flexibility of certain long bones, and the radius and ulna are textbook examples of that. They are normally somewhat flexible and thus bendable, but this was way beyond the norm. The radius and ulna were both so spongy and bendable that it was startling. I also felt very little energy in these bones. I could feel the trauma of the fall in the deadness of the bones.

I gingerly and carefully lifted up her right arm. I certainly didn't want to injure or irritate anything. I very gently began to do what I referred to above as "bone-bending." This means that I gently gripped her forearm bones, with one hand just below the elbow and one just above the wrist. I pulled my two hands apart in order to create traction between them and then I gently bent the bones a small amount in the direction that had least flexibility during the evaluation. This process creates an energetic flow in the bone that helps return it towards more normal function.

As I put some torque on the bones in her right forearm and held that position, the effect was amazing to her. It was as if the bones and the whole arm were saying, "This is perfect, do more of that." The position and touch felt extremely good to Nancy even though the pressure was very light. It felt extremely good to me, too. I was trying to think of a metaphor to describe what I felt and all I could come up with was a metaphor that was the opposite – when you take hard ice cream out of the freezer and then you wait a while (or use the microwave), and the ice cream gets softer and more pliable and takes on a totally different consistency. Only this is the opposite of what the bones felt. They started out as overly soft and pliable and as we did the traction and rotation, they gradually got more and more solid.

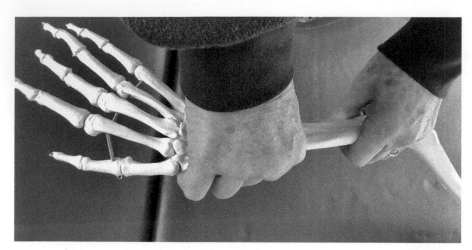

Fig. 21.1
Bone bending with the radius and ulna.

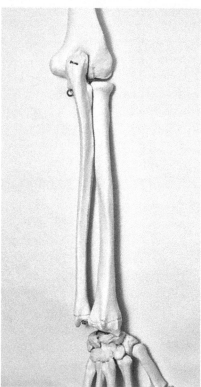

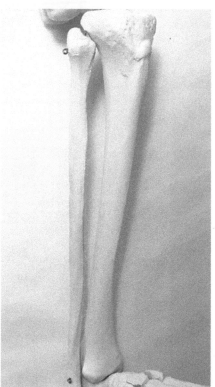

Fig. 21.2
Photo of the radius and ulna – long, thin bones of the forearm which are ideal for bone-bending.

(Photo: James McCormick.)

Fig. 21.3
Photo of the tibia and fibula – long bones of the lower leg which are also good for bone-bending.

(Photo: James McCormick.)

The bones literally changed their consistency. The feeling of Gumby-ness was reduced. We were both amazed by how good it felt, how little pressure was needed and how much change occurred. I was doing the lightest touch I could. The bones didn't want or need to be coerced or forced to do anything. That had already happened during the fall. I wanted to allow them the opportunity to move on their own, and not to force them. They responded beautifully.

I worked next on her elbows. Again a very light touch made huge changes in her elbow's range and quality of motion, as well as huge changes in her shoulder rotation. I tested the range of motion in her shoulders after the work on her forearm and elbow, and it was now normal, before I had done anything directly to her shoulder. And another remarkable thing was happening. Not only had the work made significant changes in her wrist, forearm, elbow and shoulder, the work had also made changes in Nancy. She began to feel very young. She physically collapsed, letting her torso sag and lean to the right side, no longer trying to hold herself up. As soon as she started to sag, her elbows (which I was working on at that time) got even better. Letting herself go physically (rather than holding a stiff upper lip, so to speak) let all parts of her release and relax.

As she relaxed, I could add even more rotation to the elbow joint, which allowed more change. Usually in ZB I hold these fulcrums for three to ten seconds, but these I held for minutes, following the rotation in her body. This process is called "unwinding." Nancy was very comfortable with this. She was no longer feeling out of touch with herself, but more connected to her sensations and emotions, as if getting herself back. She returned to being her strong, confident self and less her injured, weak, unsure, disconnected self. It was quite amazing how much the change in her arm changed her. And that changed her perception

of herself. Her forearm now felt strong and solid, and so did she.

At this point I still hadn't worked on her wrist, the original presenting problem. So I moved on to work there and again huge changes in the range of motion occurred with these fulcrums. These were simple fulcrums, holding steady traction with my hands above and below the wrist and then bending the wrist in different directions, based on what I felt in the joint.

The hand had started out not looking like a normal hand. It had been distorted, out of alignment and very swollen on the inside. By the end of the session it looked much more like her other hand, with less swelling and the radius much more in the right alignment. The range of motion in her wrist was better, and she had less discomfort. All of this was accompanied by more change in her torso. She felt the effects in her whole body and in her core. She kept feeling more and more connected to her power. All of this brought up some tears and sadness at what she had been through, as well as some joy at rediscovering her strength.

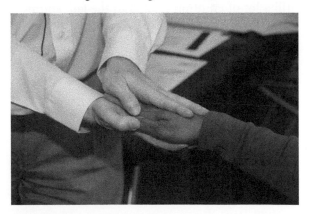

Fig. 21.4
Soothing fulcrum to the whole hand and wrist.

(Photo: Tom Gentile.)

By the end of the session she felt very happy. Her right arm was much closer to normal. She no longer wanted to collapse. Her eyes were bright and she was feeling strong and like herself. We did similar work on her left hand and though it was not as globally powerful, it was very helpful to that arm as well.

We did a second session the week after, where there was more of the same, and again she came out better in body, mind and spirit.

The third session was one week later. Nancy came in feeling much better from the first two sessions. The swelling in her right wrist was less and the motion better. The radius and ulna were much more in place. Her whole right arm looked and felt more normal. Her left arm was hardly bothering her at all.

Nonetheless, after she gave me that update, she held up her right wrist and flexed it forward part way and immediately got tears in her eyes. She said, "Whenever I bend my wrist I get sad."

A great lesson here – even though her wrist and arm were physically much better, there was still a lot of emotion related to the fall, and possibly from earlier in her life, triggered by the fall and the subsequent recovery period. One of the major tenets of Zero Balancing is to treat the whole person, regardless of where the injury is. When we do a full ZB session, we always include the whole body, not just the area of discomfort. We find this produces the most health and well-being in the person and lasts the longest. But we also pay attention to the person's emotions and how the injuries are impacting her moods and healing.

So I paid close attention to what she was saying and how much it was affecting her. We talked a while about the sadness and what it meant to her before I looked at her wrists. Then I re-evaluated her right wrist. The physical form was so much better. I also found that her range of motion was improved but still less than it should have been in both flexion and extension.

I put her arm down and let her wrist and arm rest on my hand. The arm resting there felt good and right to both of us. Even though this was non-verbal I could tell how good it felt to her and how much she wanted comfort, support and non-judgmental touching. I could feel her whole body shifting and letting go just from that contact. I was aware of how much it meant to her.

As I kept letting her arm rest on my hand, Nancy started talking. She talked for 10–15 minutes with a lot of sadness and a lot of crying. She was feeling embarrassed that she was crying and saying so much. She was feeling guilty, as if somehow she was at fault for how she felt. I continued the gentle touch of her arm resting on my hand the whole time she was talking.

She talked about her childhood and her father and how incompetent she felt, and how he reinforced that feeling. As a child she had tried to put on a brave front to compensate. I asked her if she wanted to go more into the feelings of sadness, and she hesitated. She looked uncomfortable and pained at the thought. Nonetheless she reluctantly said she would. I started to ask her to go into her body and see what she felt, and again she hesitated, but then started to try to do it. Because of her two hesitations, I stopped her. I asked her to really check in and see what she (and her body) wanted. I didn't want her to do what I wanted her to do or what she thought she should do (putting on the brave front). I wanted to help her get in touch with what she really wanted.

She took a good while to listen to herself and hear what she wanted. Finally, she said she "just wanted to be taken care of and have my arm taken care of." She didn't want to spend more time going into the sad feeling at this moment. This was not easy for her to say and was actually a breakthrough for her to say what she wanted and not what she thought looked good or seemed the right thing to others. I appreciated her for taking the time to listen to herself and totally supported her decision.

I began to work on her again. I found the right elbow was way better than before in range and quality of motion, but still less flexible than her left elbow. As I balanced her elbow joint with ZB, she began to feel more connected to herself again. She also felt a reaction in her torso of more relaxation and positive energy. I then worked on her forearm, holding it lightly with good contact. She got more and more in touch with what she felt in her body. She could let down and "collapse," as she had done in the first session. This was important for her, contradicting a pattern of needing to look competent and together and okay.

She felt so much better letting down and allowing the feeling of contact to her core. She was still sad, but as we went along that shifted. She came into greater awareness of her core self, updating her view of herself to recognize how competent she really was. I said she may not be competent to send a rocket to Mars, but she was competent in many ways. We even joked that maybe she could be competent enough to send a rocket to Mars if that was her wish. So by then we were laughing more and both feeling very engaged. She was way more at home in herself and feeling much more at ease.

She had been sitting up all this time, while I was working on her arms, so I asked her to lie back on the table to do ZB on her upper back and neck and shoulders. This part of the Zero Balancing session helped free her up over all, which also helped her

arms heal more fully and more quickly. The ZB felt good to her and let her drop even deeper into a state of relaxation and peace.

At the end of this session, Nancy slowly came back to sitting. She felt at ease and grateful. She told me how much her experience meant to her and how our connection was important to her. I told her it was meaningful and important to me as well, and that helping her get to her core also helped me feel my core, which was absolutely true.

It's an important principle to acknowledge both to myself and to clients that I also gain from working with them. When a client really opens up and moves to a liberated space, I usually feel some liberation in myself. I feel totally engaged and intensely focused, and I come out of the session more enlivened and energized.

This session felt easy to do. As Nancy tuned into her body sensations, she was able to allow the energetic changes to happen. Also, very little pressure was needed in the fulcrums. The session was much more about connection than about force or trying to make something happen. Nancy had been trying to MAKE things happen and to force things to happen her whole life. She needed to LET things happen.

We had a follow-up session a month later. Her right wrist was doing much better. It had gradually improved in strength, size, alignment and appearance. It looked much more like a normal hand and arm. It was now possible for her to hold herself up on her palms, which had not been possible before. She was more able to do her work, and she was feeling very good about that.

In this session, she asked more for help on her left neck and the trapezius muscle on her shoulder, rather than her wrist. She had been feeling sore and tight there, maybe from overworking it while trying to protect her wrist. Nonetheless I started checking her right wrist and elbow first, and the right elbow was still restricted on both internal and external rotation. It was only 25% as restricted as it had been in the beginning, but still stiff enough that it warranted more treatment.

I treated the elbow first and it noticeably improved. I then evaluated her wrist. The range of motion and the quality of motion were both much better than they had been. Flexion of the wrist joint was almost normal. The extension was still limited to 60–70% of what it should be, but that was a considerable improvement.

I gently put in the fulcrum for the wrist, compressing my fingers together above and below the wrist joint, and then separating my fingers and thumbs to create traction in the joint. This puts traction on the ligaments, which moves more energy through them and thus helps them heal. While doing the fulcrum, we got a very nice "click" in the joint, which both of us could hear and also feel. This happened when the bones adjusted. Immediately Nancy felt this was an important moment. Her wrist felt significantly better to her right away.

When I went back to evaluate, there was more range of motion and the joint looked much more "normal," with even less swelling and better alignment. Nancy felt a big change in how her wrist felt and moved. At the same time, she once again experienced a shift in herself as well. She began to allow herself to "collapse" again. She was able to let her body behave as it wanted, which was really more relaxing than collapsing. This brought some sadness to the fore again, though with few tears this time, as a lot of that had been worked through.

We talked more about her childhood, and she once again mentioned how her father always questioned her competence, and how the family dynamics led her to question her own self-worth. She felt she had to work very hard so she could see herself as competent and have others see her that way. This meant having to hold herself in a certain way and be a certain way. She never felt able to just let herself go and live from her core. It was amazing once again to see how much this pattern was tied into her hands and her response to her injuries.

I then had her lie down on the table, and we did the rest of a ZB session starting with her upper back and neck, where she had felt the pain coming into the session. As we worked she began to feel more solid in her abdomen, where weakness had resided earlier. When she checked in there now, she felt more of her own strength and her own core. I think she felt more able trust herself and her worth. It was lovely to see, and I think she felt lovely.

At the end of the session, Nancy was still lying down and I was sitting next to her. I just held her hand and wrist in my hands as gently and warmly as I could, with love and tenderness in the touch.

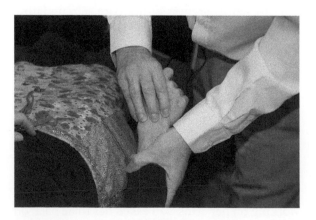

Fig. 21.5
Fulcrum to the wrist joint.

(Photo: Tom Gentile.)

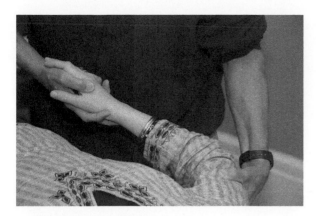

Fig. 21.6

Fulcrum to the whole arm.

(Photo: Giovanni Pescetto.)

This was similar to how I had held her hand during the last session, but I was sensing a different quality in her. She was needing the holding less though still enjoying it. It helped her to feel met, seen, supported and respected; and that was moving to us both. It felt as if her wrist and hand relaxed more, and she relaxed more into the feeling of living from her core self and not from her ideas of herself, or her family's ideas of her.

We ended the session with a general fulcrum through her whole arm to integrate all the work we had done.

This felt lovely to her. We did some closing fulcrums to end the process, all of which felt wonderful to her.

Part Four

Transformation

4

Chapter 22
Zero Balancing and the Power of Transformation

My editor, Michelle Blake, is a long time receiver and appreciator of Zero Balancing. She and her husband have taken two ZB classes so they could work with each other using Zero Balancing. We jointly decided it would be interesting and useful for me to give her a ZB session and for each of us to write down our thoughts and experiences of the process. We did the session in January 2019, as I finished the book. Michelle's version comes first below, and I have written up my notes and impressions, which follow. This session is another vivid example of the power of Zero Balancing to effect deep personal change for the client through working with the energy and structure of the bones.

As Jim and I finished the final edit of the book, I had a ZB session with him. I live in Vermont, a couple of hours away from Cambridge, but I had planned a short visit to Boston and decided to see if Jim had time to meet, because I had a lot going on in my body and spirit.

One year earlier, I'd had a malignant polyp removed, along with a series of follow-up procedures. At the time of this session with Jim, I had been free of the cancer for a year, and my mind wanted to think of it as behind me. My body did not.

Also, just before the visit to Cambridge, my husband and I had been in a significant car accident – our car had slid down a long hill, covered in black ice, on our dirt road, slammed into the embankment and ricocheted back onto the road. The front end of the car was torn up, and we were both shaken, but fine. Afterward, every time I reached the crest of that hill and headed down, I could feel my body tense up and a kind of haze settle over me along with the internal message "I am not here, this is not happening."

And somehow, in the internal logic that is barely apprehensible and often incomprehensible, my body had decided all these elements were connected — the cancer, the series of procedures, the accident and, of course, my 15-month scan that was coming up shortly after the trip to Cambridge.

My fear began to focus on the scan with the concern that this time it would not be clear. I feared I would be back where I started a year ago. I had no evidence, no symptoms, and in fact my energy and health had been noticeably improving over the year. But the fear persisted. I was feeling it quite clearly when I walked into Jim's office.

In addition, I had been going through a series of shifts in my attitude toward my work. We had moved up to Vermont just over ten years earlier, in order to write full time. Over the years, the practice of getting up, making a pot of Golden Milk tea and going to my study every morning began to effect a change, water over rock. I became more devoted to and determined about my work. I returned to writing poetry full time, something I hadn't done since I was in my twenties. My schedule became an exercise in allowing as little as possible to interfere.

I continued publishing non-fiction and began to publish poetry as well. I was writing fluently and completely taken up by the work. But when it came to finishing and publishing a manuscript, I ran into something old and implacable — my resistance to being visible. My terrible fear of being seen.

Why I feel this is not a mystery. I grew up in a series of alcoholic households, all volatile and unpredictably violent. Being the good child, visible only when it was safe, had been my mode of survival.

Also, a friend told me recently that it is often hard for adults, especially adults from homes like mine, to outstrip their parents. Which is to say, there's a set of coded messages in these families about how much success is allowed — enough to reflect well on the family, but not enough to outshine anyone.

I've been a grown-up a long time, and I often feel sick to death of my past. But being tired of it doesn't make it go away. When I went to see Jim, I had become aware of a kind of block, a big square barrier between myself and publication, especially publication of the poems, where my heart and blood, sweat and tears reside.

I have published three novels, a book of poems and a collaboration on another book, taught at Stanford and Tufts, and published poems and essays in The New York Times, Tin House, Ploughshares and other places. But I am still noticeably bad at following up when invited to submit, or keeping alive a connection with an editor who has taken my work. When an opportunity turns to look at me, I turn away. Or approach sideways, crablike.

A smart man once told me I needed to face my work head on. "Literally," he'd said. "Like when you're washing the dishes, square your hips to the sink. Or lifting something. Or writing, or sending out work, or making connections. Face front." This is good advice.

I told Jim all of this, which took a while. I was aware of time passing. We had decided to squeeze work on the book and the ZB session into his only open hour for that day, so time was at a premium. Minutes were racing by as I talked. But I stayed with it and told him as much as I could about this swirl of stuff going on in my body and psyche.

I've been working with Jim for a long time, so the basic ZB protocol is familiar and comfortable. Also, while editing the book I have learned a lot more about the potential of ZB to address exactly this set of challenges — physical, mental, spiritual, emotional, traumatic, seemingly intractable.

As soon as I finished talking, Jim asked me where I felt all this in my body. I breathed deeply a few times. My hands went to my stomach and solar plexus, the orange chakra and the yellow chakra. "Here," I said. "Also in my neck and shoulder, especially on the right side." That side of my body still has some pain and contraction from an earlier, repeated injury, though it has gotten much better over the years.

"And what does it feel like?" he asked. "Cold. Dark. Jittery. Frozen. Fast. But mostly cold and dark. And solid." There was the block — the body's pun — a solid, square, black object.

Following this we went straight to the table. After doing the usual work on my feet and legs, Jim moved to the hip bones and pelvis. He applied deep pressure to the protruding hip bones on either side, balancing them, then pushing down. After a few minutes of this, my pelvis began to feel lighter and warmer. I felt actual light inside.

When Jim began to work on my upper body, he asked me if it was okay to place his hand on the bone in the center of the chest. I said yes. I love having pressure applied to that bone, and often do it myself after yoga and meditation. As he pressed, a series of short phrases floated into my awareness.

It doesn't matter anymore.

The harm is over.

And then I heard, Goodbye, goodbye.

That last voice was light-hearted. It was flying past. It told me how to release my past. Say goodbye. So simple and undramatic, it made me smile.

I reported all this to Jim as it was happening. He asked me a question about the feelings, and I saw that though I felt light-hearted, I also had a more conscious awareness that the way I had remained connected to my family was through the harm done — done to me and to my brothers and sister. If I released that harm, I lost the connection.

I told Jim that, and then added, "But maybe because things work the way they do, if I release this connection, a new one will take its place." This made sense to him.

I'm not always so optimistic. And I don't think most people who love me would describe me as light-hearted. But there was something eerily clear about everything that was happening. It was true, and I could believe it and proceed.

After that, I became aware again of time, but it wasn't time as pressure — something I feel a lot. What arrived was a sense of time in motion, time moving through me, things moving on. It was connected to the sense that we had limited time to do this session, and we had just gotten down to work and done it. Surely the fact that I had worked with Jim for so long and had so much faith in him and his abilities, and also that I had learned so much about Zero Balancing while editing this book — all these things had opened me to whatever needed to happen.

I felt a little bit amazed. I had always assumed that any break with or acceptance of my past would have to be wrenching and dramatic. And to be clear, I've had many of those moments. But this time it was as if my psyche took care of all that — Goodbye, goodbye it said. It doesn't matter anymore. The harm is over.

I don't think this is a one-shot deal. I assume my past will reappear — or my reactions to my past will reappear — in a variety of forms. But at that moment I began walking away from harm. Which means I was walking toward health.

When I sat up, I still felt light, warm, calm. I could still hear goodbye, goodbye, and it made me laugh a little. Also, I still felt aware of time. Jim and I had done what we needed to do in an hour. Time gets smaller and larger, time moves on, moves through me. I move with it. Maybe this is what people mean by the phrase time heals.

A week later, I still hear, clearly, those phrases — It doesn't matter anymore. The harm is over. Goodbye, goodbye. I experience a sense of recognition and release. It's mild, but definite. The phrases invite me to lighten up, to have some faith, to move on, to move into what is next for me. I can stop thinking about my past if I want to. I can stop letting it be what defines me. I just finished a long poem, and this is the last section.

3. Aubade

The earth is a guide,
Follow me, she says

The white sky
as the sun rises white
at the edge of the woods

and the moon sinks into the grey blue
small brightness, clean cup

Maybe there is a third life

last green of the year
first hour of the day

What could happen
without such a past? *Anything*
says earth, *could happen*

First of all, it has been wonderful to work with Michelle. As an editor, her quality work and genuine support kept me going many times when I had felt unsure of how to proceed.

Working with her as a client with Zero Balancing has been rewarding for me, as well as for her. She has consistently over the years brought authentic and deep feelings to her sessions, which has allowed a great deal of change, both in her physical body but also personally. A lot of people who receive ZB sessions still don't know of the potential power of Zero Balancing to make a big shift in personal issues. Michelle has known this and experienced this shift from the beginning of her ZB work. I think you can see that from her write-up of her experience with this session.

This session highlights many principles of Zero Balancing that we have touched on in the book.

First of all, it illustrates the importance of having a clear, strong frame if you wish to have an empowered personal session. As we saw in Part One, Chapter 7 on *framing*, getting to a clear, concise frame helps most sessions move deeper and allows more change. Michelle came to the session wanting to work on her deep-seated fears that harked back to childhood, and while she had done much work on that part of her life, the fears were still there and had been re-triggered by recent events in her life.

To help develop the frame for the session I first listened to all that Michelle had to tell me and then asked her a few questions. Almost always when a client has a personal issue she wants to work on, one of the first things I ask is if can she feels a sensation in the body that corresponds to the issue. There are many reason for this. Having the client feel the sensation in the body shifts awareness from mentally describing what she feels to actually *experiencing* what she feels. A shamanic teacher I worked with used to say that "you cannot get from thinking to being, but you can from feeling to being." So, getting people to a feeling experience of what they are talking about is one step on the way to more dramatic change.

This process almost always leads to greater awareness for the person. She is frequently unaware of these feelings in the body and directing the client's attention gives her greater access and insight into the mind/body relationship. It also gives me a place to start looking in the body for where the energy might be held.

This verbal work with the client, and with what she feels in the body, before we go to the table, often creates a big change in itself (as we saw in Part One, Chapter 9 on the *body felt sense*). Talking honestly about strong feelings and giving the client time to feel that experience in their body often causes significant energetic shifts in the physical body and in the psyche of the client. This primes the pump and gives the session a running start. An energetic change has already taken place and this allows the body to respond even more fully to the Zero Balancing.

Often times I will use focusing techniques to help a client to keep her awareness on the bodily feelings and to tolerate the discomfort of feeling those sensations without trying to change it. Usually, if the client is able to do this, the sensations lessen just from the client bringing awareness to that part of their body.

Michelle had talked about fear in several forms so I asked where in her body she felt the fear and the "big square block." She said she felt it in her "tummy and solar plexus." My next question was, and almost always is, "and, what does it feel like?" Michelle said it felt "cold, dark, frozen, jittery, churning." Interesting that on the one hand the feeling was frozen and on the other there was also a churning experience.

With Michelle the frame we created was to lessen her fear and to help this cold, dark physical sensation to lessen. And in the process, we wanted to help her connect more deeply to her core self, which is beneath the fear and the holding.

I asked Michelle to move to the table and began the ZB session. Immediately when I put my hands on the bones in Michelle's shins I could feel in her body some of what she was talking about. There was a lot of tension in the bones and also a shakiness and unsteadiness.

These sensations were even stronger when I started to work on her lower back and pelvis – where she had felt the most fear at the beginning. There was a hardness to the tissues as if hanging on to prevent movement. There was a lack of movement, and at the same time more of that feeling of churning and shakiness. As I held gentle ZB fulcrums in the lower ribs, the lumbar area and the pelvis, these sensations began to lessen.

I felt tissues changing fairly easily and felt the energetic vibration in the area get lighter and calmer. Michelle described her own response as "feeling lighter."

As I moved to the upper body, about halfway through the session, I asked her how she was doing and she said she was doing well. I also felt the session was going well but I was still looking for something more. I felt that more change was possible and I was looking for where in the upper body the energy might be most held. The initial work on the upper body was similar to the lower body. There was still a great deal of tension in the posterior ribs and I could still feel the anxiety in this part of her body. I did all of the usual fulcrums on the upper body, which includes the posterior ribs, trapezius, the scapula, and the head and neck. All of these led to continual and gradual openings, relaxations, and more positive energetic movement.

Nonetheless, I still felt that something more was needed. I felt there was still a lot of undischarged emotion and a need to help Michelle feel more connected to the deeper parts of herself and to her core.

I began to evaluate the state of anterior ribs. There are several acupuncture points in this area of the body, on the kidney meridian, that the ancient Chinese believed had a strong effect on the spirit. The 25th point on the kidney meridian is named the Spirit Storehouse. I thought this might help Michelle connect to her deeper self and to her core. As I worked on those ribs, the effects were useful, but I began to be called by the sternum. We look at the sternum in Zero Balancing as the bony expression of the energy of the heart. We believe, and have experience to support the idea, that by working on the sternum we can help the person connect with that deep part of themselves which is said in Chinese medicine to be another "storehouse of our spirit."

Working with this bone is often a powerful part of a session and often produces large changes in the energetic field and in the person's experience.

In this case I put my hand on Michelle's sternum with light pressure but with as much connection as I could bring to it. I was aware of the warmth of the connection and then of a big shift in Michelle – her body got softer, her field got both warmer and more expanded. Her breathing got easier. The tension and shaking that was there earlier receded. I could feel a really nice shift happening. I didn't know her internal experience until she told me, but I knew something profound was happening.

She described after the session what was happening for her internally at that time – being able to say goodbye to her way of holding on to her past. She said she heard the phrases, *It doesn't matter anymore. The harm is over.* She said to me, "I don't need this anymore," meaning she didn't need to keep holding her past in the same way.

She described this as giving her feeling of "a sense of time in motion, time moving through me, things moving on." I experienced it as energy moving more freely in her body – as the tissues getting lighter and more vibrant and with more energetic juice. The big square block was gone. The shaking, quaking energy was gone.

When she sat up after the session she felt "light, warm, calm and with a bit of a laugh." To me she looked relaxed, lit up, present, with eyes clear. We were both very happy with all that had happened. I was even more glad to receive her write-up later in the week and see that she was still feeling the positive effects and had written such a beautiful poem about the possibilities now open to her.

We believe in Zero Balancing that past unprocessed hurts and traumas lead to deep-seated holding in the body and particularly in the bones. Some of these hurts, and also our early conditioning from childhood, lead to beliefs that are not necessarily in accord with the way the world is now.

Michelle realized during this process that she had unconsciously stayed connected to her family through her whole life by keeping an awareness of the harm done to her and her siblings. She had long held the erroneous and unconscious belief that "if she released the harm, she would lose the connection" to family.

When the energetic holding in the body is met in the right way, the held energy can be freed up, and not only the body can change, but also the long-held thoughts and beliefs can change. We say that the person's nervous system is updated or her perspective on herself and her life is updated to what is true in the present. She can have a more accurate view of her own capabilities and of the truth as it is now.

For Michelle these updates and realizations came spontaneously in the form of the phrases, *It doesn't matter anymore, the harm is over, Goodbye, goodbye.* This kind of shift happens spontaneously and unconsciously. They were not sought consciously by Michelle or myself. There was no intention for this to happen. I think this is a perfect example of the positive way that ZB can impact held energy or held trauma – by freeing the energy in the bones (in this case the sternum) the body/mind is free to experience the same things in a very different way. And this can have a huge effect on the person and on her life moving forward.

What could happen
without such a past? Anything
says earth, could happen

Part Five

Research on Zero Balancing

Chapter 23
Research on Zero Balancing

Over the years there have been numerous looks at how to research Zero Balancing to document its effects. This effort has been more concentrated recently. Here is a look at four very different methods of research into Zero Balancing.

Quarry and King (eds) (2016)

This book was groundbreaking. As one of the early steps on the journey of scientific inquiry into Zero Balancing, it helped lead the way to more specific research protocols. The authors, Veronica Quarry and Amanda King, are both experienced Zero Balancers. Quarry is a physical therapist, has been a practitioner of Zero Balancing for seven years and has a history as a research associate in cardiology at Tufts Medical School. King is a certified Zero Balancer and a faculty member of the Zero Balancing Health Association since 2010.

Their overarching goal was to begin the process of documenting through case histories the many benefits to people receiving Zero Balancing sessions. Quarry in particular was familiar with case studies as a valid approach to qualitative research in health care through her earlier work at Tufts.

From the start, Dr Fritz Smith, founder of ZB, and the practitioners who followed, observed and recorded histories of their patients. These informal case studies were the building blocks we used to analyze and understand our work. Quarry and King collected this information in one place for the first time, and in the process they helped lay the foundation for future research into the effects of Zero Balancing. A lot of the case studies in their book are very similar in flavor to the case histories in this book.

Quarry and King (2016) say in the introduction to their book, "Since the early 1970s practitioners and recipients of ZB have routinely experienced the many ways this modality enhances health and wholeness. This suggests the validity of the modality but scientific inquiry requires appropriate, systematic documentation to support this."

The book includes 25 case histories from certified Zero Balancing practitioners that give evidence of the broad range of effects possible from

Zero Balancing sessions, from the physical to the emotional and spiritual.

Types of case histories

The titles of the case histories vary from "Chronic pain from old injuries," to "Relief from vertigo," to "Transforming childhood abuse trauma," to "Deepens the Spiritual Direction Experience." Quarry and King (2016)

Quarry and King suggest that ZB is useful for, and applicable to, a wide range of situations. This is not widely known, even in the health care professions, and this book begins to address that lack of knowledge. In the process, Quarry and King provide encouragement to the rest of the ZB community to continue a scientific exploration of Zero Balancing.

Zero Balancing Touch Foundation – Research Pilot Studies

Research into Zero Balancing took a jump forward with the founding of the non-profit Zero Balancing Touch Foundation ("ZBTF".)

ZBTF Mission

The ZBTF is "dedicated to promoting the therapeutic use of skilled touch as a means of improving a person's health and vitality." (Zero Balancing Touch Foundation, 2015) The main aims of the ZBTF are to support education, research, and conferencing on transformational approaches to skilled touch internationally.

Research into the effects of Zero Balancing became one of the top priorities of the ZBTF, and because of its non-profit status, the Zero Balancing community was, for the first time, able to raise funds to support these research plans. As shown and explored in this book, Zero Balancing has specific, foundational theories about the effects of energy in the body. These include the idea that energy is a working tool; that energy and structure are two different but related parts in the body; that we can say we have two bodies – one of structure and one of energy; that many clients have deep meditative and altered state experiences during or after a Zero Balancing session; and that the energetic function of the bones and foundation joints in the body are very important and little understood. These have all developed over time from individual experience and observation.

Goal of research

The ZBTF board wanted to explore questions like, How much of what we see happening can be measured?, and, If measured, what new information would we find about what was happening in the body during a ZB session?

The board of directors of the ZBTF was therefore delighted when in 2015 the ZBTF was able to set up what turned out to be a series of pilot studies led by Stuart Reynolds and James Strickland of the Neuro Synchrony Institute in Austin, Texas, to attempt to measure and document the benefits of Zero Balancing sessions and to give us further insight into what might be happening to the physiology of a client when experiencing a ZB session.

The Neuro Science Institute is a highly regarded research institute with expertise in assessment, clinical practice and research methodology.

A quote from one of their reports to the ZBTF gives a glimpse into their thought processes about their contact with the Zero Balancing community.

NSI statement

The Neuro Synchrony Institute was established to bridge the gap between behavioral and physiological research in real world settings. Those activities have brought us into contact with a variety of different groups, but few more interesting than those involved with the Zero Balancing Touch Foundation. We began researching the practitioners and clients of Zero Balancing in 2015 (Strickland and Reynolds, 2017) and that has continued through 2020.

The following information on these studies is a bit technical and may contain more detail than the average lay reader cares to pursue. It is very possible to skim this section and get the main points, while for those who want more detail on the research protocols it is included here.

Held at the Lauterstein-Conway School of Massage, the researchers collected physiological data in a series of studies from 2015 to 2019. All the studies were done with wireless wrist sensors on both the ZB clients and ZB practitioners before and during each session. "NSI used unobtrusive methods with wearable technology designed by MIT (Empatica E4 and Affectiva Q) to take detailed physiological measures of both ZB practitioners and clients. This study measured electrodermal (EDA)/skin conductance changes, heart rate, heart rate variability, temperature, blood volume pulse and movement of the client and therapist. Electrodermal activity is believed

to accurately isolate sympathetic responses and differentiate emotional states (Henriques et al, 2013). NSI has extensive experience in using this instrumentation." (Strickland and Reynolds, 2017) The measurements were then analyzed looking for intriguing interactions. Simultaneously, each session was videotaped to compare what was recorded by the wrist sensors with what was being done on the client.

In these ZB research studies, "EDA measures were used in the same way as a standard polygraph test. A polygraph test measures and records several physiological indices such as blood pressure, pulse, respiration and skin conductivity or Electro Derma Activity (EDA). The underlying principle is an increase or decrease in stress will show up in these measures." (Zero Balancing Touch Foundation, 2017)

In addition, in the last two studies in the series, discussed below, tools for measuring EEG readings on both the clients and practitioners were used as well as the wrist sensors.

The first project in 2015 was a preliminary investigation working with only four participants, mostly to determine if the equipment (sensors) were able to perform up to their usual standards with the movement that is a necessary part of a ZB session. The major conclusion was a resounding yes. It was feasible to use the polygraph type technology to map the responses to a Zero Balancing session. Much of what Zero Balancers had observed for years during their ZB sessions, and some of the basic ZB principles described in this book, seemed to be visible in the physiological data that the researchers collected.

The graphs of the EDA recordings for the sessions seemed to indicate a connection where the client and practitioner came into balance or synchrony with one another based on the measurements of the sympathetic nervous system activation of both of them.

You can see this in Figure 23.1 below, where the lower lines on the graph are measurements of the Zero Balancer's activation and the upper lines are the measures of that of the client. The thick vertical line is when the session starts. The left to right scale is time and the up and down scale records the level of nervous system activation, so a lower line on the graph indicates a calmer person.

You can see the ZBer's graph moving towards that of the client seemingly to connect with the client. Shortly after the beginning of the session, their levels of activation come together and they stay together for the remainder of the session.

"The NSI report on this study says the "data strongly suggests a powerful synchronicity with the client coming into balance as they experience the skilled touch of the practitioner… the interaction between client and practitioner in a ZB session has an unusually high degree of synchrony compared to other interactions between individuals we have studied in other professional settings." (Strickland and Reynolds, 2018).

One of the main principles in this book, and indeed in all conscious touch modalities, is that ideally the practitioner will connect strongly to the client. In my original acupuncture training, Dr Worsley used to call this establishing "rapport." In Zero Balancing we call it donkey–donkey touch (see Chapter 2, Structure and Energy: Listening for the Donkey). Touching energy and structure simultaneously, the practitioner is able to connect to a deep and instinctual part of the person. This touch is always coupled with the practitioner keeping his awareness at *interface* (see Chapter 5, Living in the Moment). By keeping our awareness at the boundary where our hands meet the client's body, we keep both a clear boundary and a deep connection. The early, preliminary results of this study seemed to show the effects of these principles at work

The last major finding from this study is also observable in Figure 23.1. The ZBer and the client both got quieter and quieter as the session went on and their activation levels stayed together for the remainder of the session. Thus it was possible to record a physiological measure of the deep resting state the client often drops into during a ZB session. This is a process observed frequently

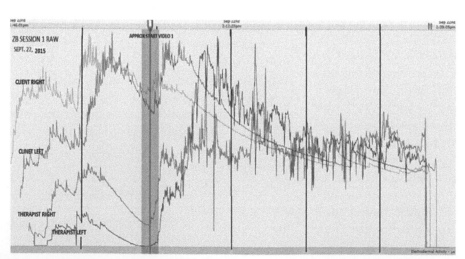

Fig. 23.1

The lower lines on the graph are measurements of the Zero Balancer's activation and the upper lines are that of the client.

(From Strickland and Reynolds, 2018.)

by all practitioners of Zero Balancing and can often lead to both general relaxation and the kind of deep transformational states we describe as an altered state of consciousness (see Chapter 10, Altered States of Consciousness).

A second, more in-depth, research study also took place in Austin, Texas in 2017. The research team again included James Strickland and Stuart Reynolds of the Neuro Synchrony Institute along with seven Zero Balancers, including Dr Fritz Smith, MD, and other faculty from the US and UK.

The first pilot study had shown that the wrist sensors used by NSI in many other settings (such as measuring mother–child interactions and giving lie detector tests) also produced valid results during ZB sessions. So a larger and more formal study was undertaken to "better understand some of the objective, measurable physiological changes that occur during Zero Balancing bodywork sessions." (Strickland and Reynolds, 2017)

Thirty volunteers were recruited, some without any previous Zero Balancing experience and some who had received ZB sessions previously. They were divided randomly into two groups, one of which received a 30-minute ZB session that was followed by 20 minutes lying on the table with no treatment. The other group had the reverse experience where they had the rest time first and then the ZB session.

"Each volunteer was also asked to complete a Likert-type well-being questionnaire developed by the Zero Balancing Touch Foundation assessing their perception of changes in their mental and emotional state before and after the ZB session. The client was asked to rate themselves using a scale with six choices for each of ten questions about their feelings. The categories included questions about wellness, positive attitude in life,

happiness, anxiousness, mental clarity, harmony, pain, stress, tension, and energy level as well as space for written comments." (Strickland and Reynolds, 2018)

One of the main goals of the study was to see if there were differences in the client's experience during the ZB sessions compared to their time of just lying down on the table. The second was so see what correlation existed between recorded changes in the physiological measures and the techniques used by the ZBers, the working signs of the client (see Chapter 6, Working Signs) and the reports from the practitioners and clients of when they felt something significant was happening.

Findings of research

Here are a few of the major findings: "On average in a group of thirty clients, in one 30 minute ZB session, ZB achieved 61% reduction of stress, compared to an average of 12% reduction in stress produced by time lying on the table.

"The 61% reduction in tension was found BOTH on the physiological (more objective measures) and the client's self-reporting in the responses to questionnaires (more subjective.) Having two separate measures reporting the same change gives more credibility to the results.

"Averaging the findings for stress, tension and anxiety there was a 51% reduction in those three areas combined, based on the questionnaires. [Fig. 23.2; see Chapter 19, Anxiety and Depression]

"The positive changes recorded by the physiological measures correlate well with the times fulcrums were being applied to the clients and/or to the working signs of the clients, giving evidence that the ZB fulcrums were causing the observed changes." (Strickland and Reynolds, 2017)

Here is a list of the final conclusions from NSI from this study:

Conclusions of research

"This is one of the very few studies that takes on the challenging tasks of building the bridges between bodywork and other behavioral health disciplines. This study represents a preliminary review although we can draw the following relevant conclusions:

- Physiological changes in stress can be measured using unobtrusive wearable instrumentation

- Zero Balancing techniques and working signs are detectable in physiological data

- Physiological measures confirm client self-reports and observations that Zero Balancing is a stress reducing experience

- All participants rated Zero Balancing bodywork as a positive emotional experience from Pre-and Post-Questionnaires

- Zero Balancing markedly reduced the perception of stress, tension and anxiety

- Zero Balancing showed clients greater perceived feeling of wellness, positivity of self and others, mental clarity and harmony

- We have such compelling data that it should be shared with others in the healing and health professions." (Strickland and Reynolds, 2018)

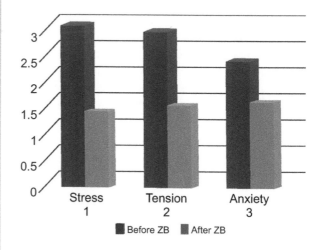

Perceived Stress, Tension and Anxiety Before and After ZB

Before ZB / After ZB

Fig. 23.2

This shows participants' perception of the effects of ZB sessions on their experience of stress, tension, and anxiety.

(From Strickland and Reynolds, 2018.)

One of the most interesting pieces of information from the study only came to our awareness after looking at the data on the graphs. In one session a dish was dropped resulting in a loud clatter. The Zero Balancer clearly heard the noise consciously and their EDS readings reflected how startled they were, showing up as a large spike in the graph of the activation state of the practitioner. The remarkable result in this session was that not only did the client did not have any conscious awareness of hearing the noise, but the graph of the reactivity of the client demonstrated no "startle" response. So not only did the client not hear the noise consciously, it seems as if their unconscious was not aware of it either. They showed no change in their EDA. In Figure 23.1 you can see at one point the line for the practitioner spike strongly and quickly, which was when the noise happened. The practitioner EDA showed a startle. If you look at the line in the graph for the client you can see that the client's EDA registered no change at all.

This led to contemplation of why that would be true. When coupled with the significant reduction of stress, this suggests ZB facilitates a form of expanded state of consciousness for the client. In an expanded state of consciousness (see Chapter 10), a person's awareness is not limited to the present reality and people often have their attention focused inside, and are not aware of the outside world. This may have been what was happening.

There was one last major piece of this study. During the same visit to Austin, the researchers began preliminary exploration of the possibility of achieving accurate EEG readings on the clients receiving Zero Balancing sessions. Two very limited EEG studies were completed with the subjects wearing different special headgear with numerous sensors to record EEG measurements of the brain waves during ZB sessions. One set

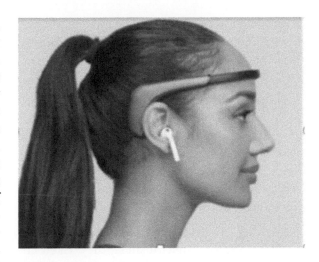

Fig. 23.3

Headgear used to record EEG measurements during ZB sessions.

(From Strickland and Reynolds, 2018.)

of headgear (Fig. 23.3) with fewer leads proved be much more useful for this type of study. It allowed both the practitioner and the client to have their heads moved and still get accurate EEG measurements.

EEG measures taken during two trial sessions suggested two things: (1) the headgear required to measure EEG activity can function well for both the practitioner and the client during a ZB session; (2) ZB seemed to facilitate a deep change in brain patterns being observed on the monitors. Initial evidence indicated a change in brain waves where the subject dropped into deeper states during a ZB session that are different from those manifest during a rest period.

These results led the Zero Balancing Touch Foundation Board to authorize a further study with the objective of exploring ZB's effect on brain behavior; that is, to explore whether ZB facilitates expanded states of consciousness by reading EEGs of both patient and practitioner during ZB sessions. This study was done in November 2018, also in Austin, and led to several interesting findings.

NSI found that when the wrist sensors of the EDA indicated reduction of tension in the client, the EEG reading of the brainwave patterns were also indicating the same kind of tension reduction. "What we detected in one type of measure was frequently detectable in the other measures." (Strickland and Reynolds, 2018)

Looking for evidence of expanded states or altered states of consciousness, they asked clients after the session at which points during the session they felt they were in an expanded state. The researchers then looked at both the EDA and EEG measures at those times in the sessions and found that "both readings were very different from the readings at other times in the sessions. There seemed to be physiological markings of when the client was in an expanded state of awareness." (Strickland and Reynolds, 2018)

Figure 23.4 (from the 2017 study) also shows physiological evidence of what looks like an expanded state at the end of a session where the extended reduction in the tension shown lasts a long time. This coincides with both a time of extreme quiet in the client and the client observing later that they were having a very deep experience.

One unexpected result showed up: the brainwaves taken when one client was asked to recount her experience of the session, while still hooked up to the EEG instruments, were strikingly similar to what her brainwaves had been during the actual experience. The recollection of the procedures gave almost the same experience as the actual experience.

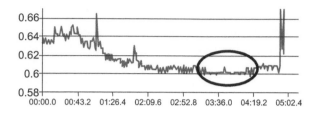

Fig. 23.4

The x-axis shows time and the y-axis shows measurement of stress levels. Lower stress levels are shown where the line on the graph dips. The lowest segment on the graph (bottom right) lasts a long time with little movement when compared to other parts of the graph, showing a very quiet state for the client.

(From Strickland and Reynolds, 2018.)

The remarkable synchrony between client and practitioner we had seen in the earlier studies continued to show up in this study.

The information gained from these studies is still being analyzed and there is hope it will be more widely available in the near future.

Rhoads, Murphy, Doucette and Gentile (2020)

The final results of this study were still being analyzed at the publication deadline for this book. What is included here is a preliminary report. For the full study go to https://thekeep.eiu.edu/ijzbtt/vol1.)

The research efforts of the Zero Balancing community have gradually become more sophisticated. This pilot study was the first to measure the effects of Zero Balancing sessions over time, and it was the first to include both quantitative and qualitative measures. The research was carried out under the auspices of Eastern Illinois

University, and overseen by Professor Misty Rhoads, a long-time EIU faculty member specializing in public health and research methods. The final results of the study are still being analyzed at this time, so this is a partial report.

The study is particularly significant because it captures both qualitatively and quantitatively the full range of Zero Balancing effects. It documents both with numbers and with words the client's experiences across a wide variety of situations. Even though this was a pilot study, the goals were ambitious. The main goal was to explore and document the effects of ZB on all aspects of wellness: "the physical, mental, emotional and spiritual dimensions of wellness." (Rhoads et al, 2020)

The results show clearly that these ZB sessions did, in fact, affect the participants in all of these ways (see Chapter 21, Unifying Body, Mind, and Spirit).

Four clients each received Zero Balancing sessions once a week for four weeks from certified Zero Balancing practitioners. They were also asked to fill out a questionnaire including Likert questions and open-ended questions. At the end of the four sessions each participant was interviewed (and video recorded) to explore their experiences during the ZB sessions.

Themes of the study

"A small sampling of these themes in the quotes from the interviews: 'I am more at peace and just allowing;' 'More awareness of my entire body;' 'ZB brings me back to myself;' 'I feel woven together;' 'I have a real appreciation of how everything is connected.'" (Rhoads et al, 2020).

Qualitative responses were gathered from the open-ended questions and the interviews. The main themes that showed up through many of the interviews were the client's feelings of "integration and connection".

These comments all agree with our long understanding of the effects of Zero Balancing sessions. Zero Balancing is always a full body session. Some bodywork techniques work only on the areas of the body that have symptoms or where the client reports difficulty. Every ZB session includes working on the whole of the body. Because of that there is almost always a sense for the person of feeling unified and connected, both to the self and to the outer world. This includes not just their body but their whole being, body, mind and spirit. This study has captured this particularly well by listening to the direct words of the clients.

I was struck by this study. When I read it I had already written Chapter 12 in this book, talking about the process of using ZB to *amplify the wellness* in a client. One of the beautiful uses of ZB is to do just that. To help someone who already feels okay, or even good, to feel even better. There is a beautiful example of that with Walter in Chapter 12.

In a similar but slightly different vein, Chapter 13, Caring, Compassion, and Containment gives another example of how increase the well-being of a client who is already feeling well. This study has captured what we often say in ZB, which is "to make normal better."

The authors' conclusion of the study is important: "ZB is an effective method to increase wellness and balance in the physical, emotional, mental, and spiritual dimensions as evidenced by 100% of participants stating increased physical relaxation, mental clarity, interests in work and

Table 23.1

Other frequently cited effects of ZB sessions in the client's responses to the questionnaire and the interview (Rhoads et al, 2020).

Themes	Significant Participant Statements
Relaxation	"I don't think I have ever been this relaxed"
Decreased stress	"ZB just helps me handle stress"
Ease of movement	"More awareness of my entire body"
Emotional regulation	"I don't overreact as much"
Mental clarity and focus	"I feel mentally uncluttered"
Increased sense of personal development	"I am more joyful and appreciative of the small moments"
Body awareness	"My bones feel electrified and my whole skeletal structure seems lengthened"

friends, and feeling less controlled by external factors". (Rhoads et al, 2020)

These conclusions can be seen in Figures 23.5 and 23.6. Of particular interest is Figure 23.5, where clients say their abilities for both contemplation and imagination strongly increase after four Zero Balancing sessions. This speaks to the effects of ZB sessions being positive on the whole person, body, mind and spirit. All of the person is affected not just physical tension or physical complaints. Figure 23.6 shows the amount of physical relaxation achieved from ZB.

In one sense, for the Zero Balancer, this confirms what we already know, but for the general public this study gives strong evidence to support the anecdotal observations of the ZB practitioners.

Murphy (2019)

Mary Murphy is a senior Zero Balancing faculty member and long-time practitioner of ZB and of many other healing techniques involving conscious touch. The following is a summary of her qualitative study of the relationship of Zero Balancing to contemplative practices. The report received the approval of the Institutional Review Board of Naropa University.

While the title of this study cites education, it involves interviews of 13 members of the Zero Balancing faculty, all of whom are long-time ZB practitioners and teachers, and includes discussion of their perception of their practice of Zero Balancing as well as their teaching.

"It was my premise that cultivating our embodied awareness through contemplative practice increases our ability to teach and practice touch skills." (Murphy, 2019)

I particularly like this study as it focuses on the deeper aspects of Zero Balancing, its use for greater personal change and transformation through expanded states of consciousness, the

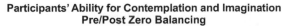

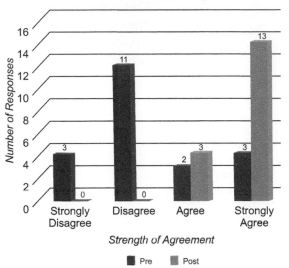

Fig. 23.5

This shows a strong increase in the ability to imagine and contemplate based on self-reports of the participants.

(From Rhoads et al, 2020.)

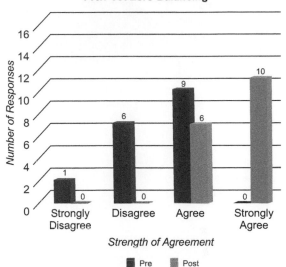

Fig. 23.6

This shows a degree of improvement in participants' perception of relaxation after ZB.

(From Rhoads et al, 2020.)

main topic of this book (see Chapter 10, Altered States of Consciousness.)

Murphy looks at what helps practitioners learn to create the conditions for their clients to have these transformative experiences. The main learning from the study is that embodied connection and contemplative practices are essential to creating these kinds of changes. "*Embodiment*, being aware of directly experiencing one's body, emotions and thoughts in the present moment, was collectively agreed upon as a pre-requisite for both bodywork teaching and practice. All 13 of the co-researchers mentioned some version of the importance of staying present in the body." (Murphy, 2019). See also Chapter 9 in this book, Body Felt Sense.

Throughout this book I have made the case that having a client learn to become more aware of their bodily sensations strongly aids their ability to have more significant results from their sessions. Murphy is saying here that the same thing is true for practitioners. If they learn to pay more attention to their own bodily sensations and their own inner experience, their work becomes more profound for their clients.

Murphy asked the practitioners a series of questions about their own use of contemplative practices, their view of how that affected their Zero Balancing, and if they saw ZB itself as a contemplative practice.

One of the main conclusions from this study might be stated as: "The first three themes,

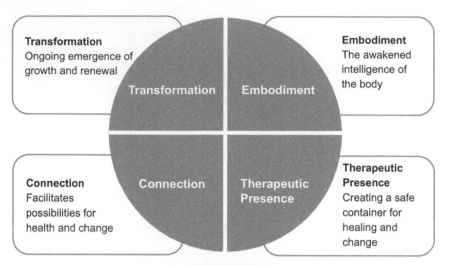

Fig. 23.7

*Embodiment >
Therapeutic Presence>
Connection >
Transformation.*

(From Murphy, 2019.)

Main themes

The main themes that emerged from the study were:

1. Embodiment – the awakened intelligence of the body

2. Therapeutic Presence – the creation of a safe container for healing and change

3. Connection – the mechanism of how engaged connection facilitates possibilities for health

4. Transformation – the on-going emergence of growth.

Every one of the respondents agree that ZB itself is a contemplative practice, and all agreed that this type of practice had a big effect on their Zero Balancing sessions. (Murphy, 2019)

Embodiment, Therapeutic Presence and Connection, need to be in place for the fourth, Transformation, to take place. This appears to me as a cycle so once the person goes through one cycle, the transformation feeds back in to growing embodiment, therapeutic presence and connection." (Murphy, 2019) This agrees completely with my main thesis in this book (Fig. 23.7).

Conclusion

The Zero Balancing Touch Foundation Board realizes we are still at the beginning of serious research into Zero Balancing and conscious touch, but we have made a significant start. There is much more work to do. The ZBTF would like to undertake and support many further research projects. We hope at some point to do more studies with NSI – such a more comprehensive study of the effects of several ZB sessions over time to compliment the 4 x 4 study. We hope to explore the effects of Zero Balancing for certain specific conditions, from improved sleep to osteoporosis. We hope to look in more detail at the EEG effects of Zero Balancing and also to see how that compares with other activities, such as the effects of massage and meditation.

Bibliography

Doucette M (2010) Waking to Eden. Wilmington, Vermont: author.

Fosha D (2000) The Transforming Power of Affect. New York: Basic Books.

Gendlin E (1978) Focusing. New York: Bantam Books.

Hamwee J (1999) Zero Balancing: Touching the Energy of Bone. London: Singing Dragon.

Henriques R, Paiva A, Attunes C (2013) Accessing Emotion Patterns from Affective Interactions Using Electrodermal Activity. A paper given at Affective Computing and Intelligent Interaction (ACII), 2013 Humaine Association Conference. Available at: www.researchgate.net/publication/261450645_Accessing_Emotion_Patterns_from_Affective_Interactions_Using_Electrodermal_Activity

Hext A (2020) Structural Energetics in Zero Balancing Bodywork. London: Singing Dragon.

Larre C and Rochat de la Vallee E (1996) The Seven Emotions. Cambridge: Monkey Press.

Levine PA Waking the Tiger: Healing Trauma (1997). Berkeley, CA: North Atlantic Books.

Maslow A (1943) A Theory of Human Motivation. Psychological Review 50:370–396.

Modell A (1993) The Private Self. Cambridge: Harvard Press.

Murphy M (2019) Cultivating Embodied Connection: The Role of Contemplative Practices in Bodywork Education. Email to J McCormick (jimmc5@comcast.net), 2019.

Quarry V and King A (eds) (2016) Experiencing the Power of Zero Balancing. Palm Beach Gardens: Upledger Productions.

Rhoads M, Murphy M, Doucette M and Gentile T (2020) Integrating Zero Balancing into the Physical, Mental, Emotional and Spiritual Dimensions of Wellness: A Mixed-Methods Pilot Study. Email to J McCormick (jimmc5@comcast.net), 2020.

Schwartz R (1995) Internal Family Systems Therapy. New York: Guildford Press.

Smith F (1986) Inner Bridges. Atlanta: Humanics New Age.

Smith, F (2005) Alchemy of Touch. Taos: Complementary Medicine Press.

Strickland J and Reynolds S (2017) Email to the Zero Balancing Touch Foundation (info@zbtouch.org), 2017.

Strickland J and Reynolds S (2018) Email to the Zero Balancing Touch Foundation (info@zbtouch.org), 2018.

Sullivan J and Smith F (eds) (2020) Core Zero Balancing Study Guide (3rd edn). Cambridge: Zero Balancing Touch Foundation.

Sullivan J (2014) Zero Balancing Expanded. Palm Beach Gardens, FL: Upledger Productions.

Vaillant L (1997) Changing Character. New York: Basic Books.

Van der Kolk B (2014) The Body Keeps the Score. New York: Viking Penguin.

Zero Balancing Touch Foundation (2015) Mission Statement of the ZBTF [online] Available at: zbtouch.org

Zero Balancing Touch Foundation (2017) NSI Research Results and Overview [online]. Available at: zbtouch.org/2017-nsi-research-results-and-overview/

Permissions

Preface

Different Types of Fulcrums used in Zero Balancing. Illustrations by Fritz Smith, used with permission of the Zero Balancing Touch Foundation.

Shimmering Light of the moon on the sea at night. Photo: Shutterstock.

Introduction

Maslow – hierarchy of needs. (See en.wikipedia. org/wiki/Self-actualization)
(Originally published in Maslow A (1943) A theory of human motivation, Psychological Review 50, 370–396.)

Author doing Zero Balancing on the upper body Photo: Tom Gentile.

Fig. 1.1
Donkey – Metaphor for touching the instinctual response by touching energy and structure simultaneously and consciously.
Photo: Ricardo Villalobos

Fig. 2.1
In Zero Balancing we use light as our model for understanding energy and structure.
Illustrations by Fritz Smith, used with permission of the Zero Balancing Touch Foundation.

Fig. 2.2
Sailboat – the Boat is the structure and the Wind is the energy.
Photo: Shutterstock.

Fig. 2.3
Sweet spot in a tennis racquet.
Photo: Shutterstock.

Fig. 2.4
Rib cage and bones of the upper body.
Photo by Kathy Plunket Versluys. Used with permission of the Zero Balancing Touch Foundation.

Fig. 3.1
All the articulations between the bones named in this photo are true foundation joints, with very small range of motion and no voluntary muscles across them.
Photo by Kathy Plunket Versluys. Used with permission of the Zero Balancing Touch Foundation.

Fig. 3.3
Pelvis showing the sacrum and the sacro-iliac joint.
Photo: Shutterstock.

Fig. 3.4
One handed half moon vector to balance the tarsal bones in the foot.
Photo: Della Watters; WattersWorks & Company.

Fig. 4.1
The bones of the pelvis and hip joint.
Photo: by Kathy Plunket Versluys. Used with permission of the Zero Balancing Touch Foundation.

Fig. 4.2
Energy moving through the bones of pelvis and hip.
Photo: Shutterstock.

Fig. 4.3
Energy flowing through a bone.
Photo: Mary Murphy, with permission.

Fig. 5.1
Vocabulary of touch – different ways of working with energy. In Zero Balancing we use interface touch.
Illustrations by Fritz Smith, used with permission of the Zero Balancing Touch Foundation.

Fig. 8.1
Half moon vector at the feet.
Photo: Tom Gentile.

Fig. 9.1
Working with the posterior rib cage in Zero Balancing.
Photo: Kathryn McNeils.

Fig. 10.1
The serenity of a client in an altered state.
Image: iStock-180829725.jpg

Fig. 10.2
Fulcrum from the hip joint and down the side of the gall bladder meridian.
Photo: Giovanni Pescetto.

Fig. 13.1
The caring hands of Dr Fritz Smith.
Photo: Giovanni Pescetto.

Fig. 13.3
Half moon vector to balance the tarsal bones in the foot.
Photo: Della Watters; WattersWorks & Company.

Fig. 16.1
The sternum, manubrium, clavicle and rib cage.
Photo: Shutterstock.

Fig. 21.4
Soothing fulcrum to the whole hand and wrist.
Photo: Tom Gentile.

Fig. 21.5
Fulcrum to the wrist joint.
Photo: Tom Gentile.

Fig. 21.6
Fulcrum to the whole arm.
Photo: Giovanni Pescetto.

Fig. 23.1
The lower lines on the graph are measurements of the Zero Balancer's activation and the upper lines are that of the client.
From Strickland and Reynolds, 2018.

Fig. 23.2
This shows participants' perception of the effects of ZB sessions on their experience of stress, tension, and anxiety.
From Strickland and Reynolds, 2018.

Fig. 23.3
Headgear used to record EEG measurements during ZB sessions.
From Strickland and Reynolds, 2018.

Fig. 23.4
The x-axis shows time and the y-axis shows measurement of stress levels. Lower stress levels are shown where the line on the graph dips.

The lowest segment on the graph (bottom right) lasts a long time with little movement when compared to other parts of the graph, showing a very quiet state for the client.
From Strickland and Reynolds, 2018.

Fig. 23.5
This shows a strong increase in the ability to imagine and contemplate based on self-reports of the participants.
From Rhoads et al, 2020.

Fig. 23.6
This shows a degree of improvement in participants' perception of relaxation after ZB.
From Rhoads et al, 2020.

Fig. 23.7
Embodiment >Therapeutic Presence > Connection > Transformation.
From Murphy, 2019.

Index

Index